FUTURESCAN™
Healthcare Trends and Implications
2018-2023

CONTENTS

Moving Ahead on the Long Road Toward Value-Based Healthcare

by Ian Morrison, PhD

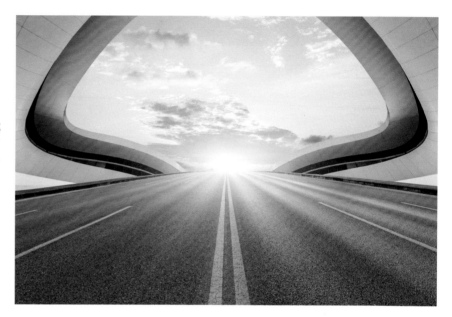

Futurescan 2018–2023 brings together an impressive lineup of guest authors who provide wide-ranging insights and perspectives on the important trends healthcare leaders must be prepared for regardless of what may happen with the ongoing twists and turns of the political and policy debates in Washington, DC. In particular, this year's *Futurescan* provides important evidence of progress regarding healthcare's long road toward value.

Reform

Mike Leavitt, former governor of Utah and former secretary of the US Department of Health & Human Services in the George W. Bush administration, draws on his vast experience to put the long-term future of healthcare payment reform in perspective.

The founder of the Leavitt Group urges hospital and health system leaders to move beyond the "fog of war" created by the current political and policy uncertainties and to focus on the shift from fee-for-service to value-based reimbursement. In Leavitt's estimation, the nation's healthcare system is 25 years into a 40-year journey on the path to value, and although progress may at times seem glacially slow, the direction is clear.

Leavitt reviews the range of payment initiatives emerging in both the public and private sectors, focusing specifically on the roles that the Medicare Access and CHIP Reauthorization Act (MACRA), Medicare Advantage, Medicaid managed care, the integration of behavioral health, and public and private accountable care organizations are playing in transforming the healthcare reimbursement landscape. While acknowledging that results to date have been modest, he emphasizes the encouraging signs that value-based payment can spur providers to improve the quality of care, reduce costs, and be more responsive to consumers.

Leavitt sums up by noting that "innovative leaders who recognize the economic imperatives mandating change . . . and engage with alternative payment and delivery models will be rewarded."

Consumerism

Richard L. Gundling, senior vice president of healthcare financial practices at the Healthcare Financial Management Association, provides an insightful perspective on the future of healthcare consumerism, pointing out that out-of-pocket costs and the process of paying for health services have become major sources of dissatisfaction for many Americans.

To address the problem, Gundling says, physicians, hospitals, and health systems must focus on developing patient-friendly billing practices that make consumers aware of their financial responsibilities for care; provide empathetic, compassionate guidance on patients' options for payment; and avoid sending surprise bills.

About the Author

Ian Morrison, PhD, is an author, consultant, and futurist. He received an undergraduate degree from the University of Edinburgh, Scotland; a graduate degree from the University of Newcastle upon Tyne, England; and an interdisciplinary doctorate in urban studies from the University of British Columbia, Canada. He is the author of several books, including the best-selling *The Second Curve: Managing the Velocity of Change*. Morrison is the former president of the Institute for the Future and a founding partner of Strategic Health Perspectives, a forecasting service for clients in the healthcare industry.

He also urges providers to pay increased attention to consumers as decision makers, given that insurers and employers are increasingly shifting to high-deductible health plans and incentivizing patients to "shop" for services. Gundling anticipates that the trend toward consumerism will only intensify "as the volume-to-value transformation picks up steam."

Cybersecurity

Cybersecurity experts John Riggi and Patrick Pilch of professional services company BDO deliver a fascinating review of the challenges online threats pose to hospitals and health systems. Recent massive cybersecurity hacks and ransomware attacks have rocked major health insurance companies and health providers across the globe, particularly in the United Kingdom and the United States.

To assist leaders in assessing their vulnerabilities and adopting best practices, Riggi, who leads BDO's cybersecurity and financial crimes practice, and Pilch, the national coleader of The BDO Center for Healthcare Excellence & Innovation, urge healthcare organizations to take the following important steps:

- Introduce cyber hygiene policies and a cybersecurity training program based on employees' roles.
- Identify and address any potential weak points in information technology systems.
- Implement threat monitoring and analytics tools capable of detecting an attack, and apply investigative and digital forensic capabilities to understand what went wrong and assess the damage.
- Develop an internal and external crisis communications plan that is aligned with an existing enterprise risk management framework.
- Make sure your organization has adequate cybersecurity insurance.

They conclude by observing that "for healthcare, a cyber attack . . . is a human safety issue. Responding quickly can be a matter of life or death. Providers have to make sure their defense measures keep pace with their technological advances—or else face the growing consequences."

Equity of Care

Eugene A. Woods, FACHE, president and CEO of Carolinas HealthCare System and immediate past chair of the American Hospital Association board of trustees, offers thoughtful insights on the link between care disparities and social determinants of health.

Woods, a passionate leader and proponent of eliminating disparities, points out that despite hospitals' and health systems' best intentions, enormous differences in healthcare quality, access, and outcomes persist because of factors of race, ethnicity, income, and geography. He goes on to stress the key role that social determinants of health play in driving disparities.

Woods lays out an impressive agenda for how providers can lead the way in addressing the problem. For example, they can use data analytics to assist with hotspotting, optimize their workforces to reflect the diversity of their communities, and seek greater collaboration with a wide range of community partners.

Woods also advises leaders to incorporate health equity goals and outcome measures into their organizations' strategic plans. He closes by stating, "A future where individuals have the chance to reach their highest potential for health regardless of where they live, what language they speak, or what they look like: That is the promising vision within our reach. With the right road map, and a firm resolve, we can make it happen."

Emergency Care

James J. Augustine, MD, a member of the board of directors of the American College of Emergency Physicians, highlights the rapid changes taking place in emergency care. He says the future of the field is being shaped by the convergence of several market forces:

- Changing consumer expectations that demand new and more affordable options for emergency and immediate care
- Pressure from both businesses and commercial and government insurers to lower medical costs
- The increasing prevalence of urgent care centers and walk-in clinics
- The emergence of new models, such as freestanding emergency departments, microhospitals, and telemedicine
- Steady growth in hospital-based emergency department volumes

Augustine advises leaders to strategically determine the most effective ways for their organizations to respond to these developments while remaining mission focused. In his words, "Hospi-

> This year's *Futurescan* provides important evidence of progress regarding healthcare's long road toward value.

tals will continue to serve as the front line and safety net for our healthcare system and the millions of Americans, both insured and uninsured, who rely on them daily for emergency care."

Facilities

Don King, lead for the Healthcare Executive Leadership Council of the American Hospital Association's American Society for Healthcare Engineering, reviews current and future trends in healthcare facilities management. The former head of facilities operations for Kaiser Permanente emphasizes the following implications for healthcare organizations:

- As capital investments shift away from the main hospital campus, an increasing number of providers are buying or renting former retail buildings to bring healthcare services closer to the community. Doing so often requires dispersed administration and facilities management, as well as duplication of services and equipment.

- The need to withstand earthquakes, floods, and other catastrophes will tax the budgets of many healthcare organizations as they make costly enhancements to strengthen their facilities.
- In this age of growing societal violence, hospital leaders need to undertake facility improvements to enhance patient and caregiver security—for example, creating control centers and safe rooms and installing automatic locking devices on doors and elevators.
- With the threat of narcotics theft on the rise, hospital and outpatient facility pharmacies must increase pharmaceutical safety, especially for drugs that are in demand on the street. That means adding more surveillance cameras, alarms, and other security equipment.

King wraps up his article by saying, "The new era of healthcare requires greater forethought and planning for hospital and health system facilities."

Role of Employers

David Lansky, PhD, president and CEO of the Pacific Business Group on Health (PBGH), provides an important perspective on the role employers are playing as a driving force in transforming healthcare delivery and reimbursement.

Lansky draws on the experience of the PBGH and its members (which include Disney, Boeing, Apple, Intel, and others) as they strive to make the nation's healthcare system more responsive to businesses and their employees, improve the quality of care, slow the escalation of medical costs, and increase the affordability of services.

He highlights the shift toward greater direct contracting with providers by self-funded employers and public purchasers of health insurance through value-based approaches that increase physician, hospital, and health system accountability. Lansky says examples such as accountable care organizations and bundled-payment models are being driven partly by employers' frustration with the lack of progress health plans have shown in addressing their concerns.

Looking to the future, Lansky provides wise counsel to providers on how they can seize opportunities with self-insured employers:

- Understand your own performance in terms of cost and quality.
- Talk to local employers.
- Redesign care to achieve continuously improved value.
- Engage in regional community efforts.

Lansky concludes by calling on businesses and providers to work together to "accelerate a national commitment to delivering greater value to patients and to society as a whole."

Provider Health Plans

Paul H. Keckley, PhD, a widely respected healthcare consultant and thought leader, sheds light on the trend toward provider-sponsored health plans (PSPs). Keckley notes the difficulties these plans face in the marketplace but also explains why many hospitals are embracing PSPs as a strategy to avoid being excluded from narrow health networks, gain insights into the pros and cons of assuming greater risk as payers move toward value-based care,

and position themselves for success in population health initiatives.

Keckley urges leaders to calibrate their PSP decisions, recognizing the inevitability that their margins will be under pressure from purchasers. He points to three potential paths moving forward:

- For hospitals that already sponsor plans, the focus will be on enrollment growth and benefit design innovation, with special attention paid to contracting opportunities in Medicaid and Medicare.
- For hospitals that are not currently offering plans but are located in markets where sponsorship makes sense, the time may be right to consider a PSP strategy.
- For hospitals in markets where sponsoring a PSP is not feasible or prudent, participation in shared-risk arrangements with payers will be an increasingly important option.

Keckley closes with the observation that although PSPs are not right for many hospitals, they are "certainly worth considering if circumstances suggest there is opportunity."

Conclusion

Futurescan 2018–2023 provides important insights into how healthcare organizations can proactively respond to key trends in the field. Of course, hospitals and health systems must continue to focus on the basics of cost management and continuous improvement in clinical care. These eternal verities will only help to advance value-based care for purchasers who demand it, for consumers who expect it, and for communities across the nation that deserve it.

The Value of Perspective

by Mike Leavitt

The phrase "fog of war" was coined by Prussian general Carl von Clausewitz in the nineteenth century. It refers to the uncertainty, confusion, and chaos that ensue during the intensity of battle. In such moments, individual pieces of information have little context, so the relevance and importance of facts or outcomes can be easily misperceived. Battle strategists reference the need for battlefield awareness and the ability to see narrow events in the context of the big picture.

A similar fog surrounds the current healthcare debate. The swirl of constant news perpetuates uncertainty and confusion. The drama of politically charged sound bites could easily cause one to lose sight of the bigger and longer-term picture.

Healthcare reform in the United States cannot be adequately understood without viewing the current debate from a broader perspective. The nation is roughly 25 years into a 40-year transformation period. The actions of the current Congress are another iteration of that ongoing process.

The Economic Mandate to Change

When we pull back and contextualize the current healthcare

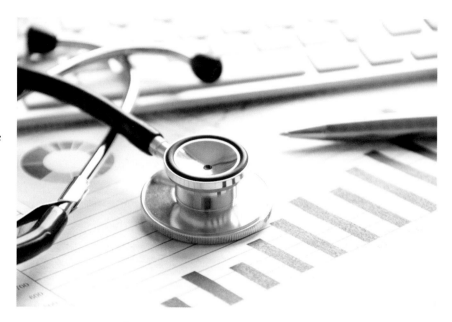

conversation, we see that an economic imperative is driving reform. Although politics dominates much of the discussion, the mandate to change healthcare is profoundly economic. Healthcare consumes an increasingly large share of the federal budget, draining money from education, national security, and other programs essential to America's present and future strength (exhibit 1). Indeed, dramatically rising medical costs compromise our economic position and threaten our leadership on the global stage.

Context also allows us to see that the economic mandate to change is not new. When Medicare and Medicaid passed into law in 1965, providing coverage to millions of older and poor citizens, many experts saw problems from the beginning. Implementing large entitlement programs in a fee-for-service system, which rewards the volume of services provided, created the wrong incentives.

In the late 1960s, professors at Yale University sought to fix the problem by means of diagnosis-related groups

About the Author

Mike Leavitt is the founder and general partner of Leavitt Partners, a healthcare intelligence business that helps clients successfully navigate the evolving role of value in healthcare. Over the course of his career, Leavitt has held substantial leadership positions in both the private and public sectors. Prior to founding Leavitt Partners, he served in two positions in the cabinet of President George W. Bush—first as administrator of the US Environmental Protection Agency (2003–2005) and then as secretary of the US Department of Health & Human Services (2005–2009). In 1993, he was elected governor of Utah, a position he held for three terms (1993–2003). He also previously served as chief executive of The Leavitt Group, a family business that is now the nation's second-largest privately held insurance brokerage. He earned a bachelor's degree in business while working in the insurance industry. His book *Finding Allies, Building Alliances* (Jossey-Bass, 2013) chronicles his expertise and passion for collaboration.

FUTURESCAN SURVEY RESULTS
Reform

How likely is it that the following will happen by 2023?

Very Likely (%)	Somewhat Likely (%)	Neutral (%)	Somewhat Unlikely (%)	Very Unlikely (%)
37	37	15	9	2

At least 10 percent of your hospital's or health system's patients will be covered by risk-based population health and bundled-payment reimbursement contracts.

71	23	3	2	1

Your hospital or health system will increase its collaboration with other providers (e.g., doctors, hospitals, post-acute care organizations) and payers on population health management as a strategy to improve clinical outcomes.

45	35	14	5	2

Your hospital or health system will increase its investment in behavioral health services at least in part to meet the requirements of Medicaid managed care programs.

27	36	23	11	4

Your hospital or health system will increase its participation in narrow health insurance networks by 25 percent as a strategy to grow patient volumes.

Note: Percentages in each row may not sum exactly to 100% because of rounding.

What Hospital Executives Anticipate by 2023

- A clear majority (71 percent) of leaders believe it is very likely they will increase collaboration with other providers and payers on population health management. Another 23 percent say it is somewhat likely.

- Eight in ten respondents (80 percent) think it is somewhat to very likely their organization will increase investment in behavioral health services, at least in part to meet the requirements of Medicaid managed care programs.

- Three-quarters (74 percent) say it is at least somewhat likely that 10 percent or more of their patients will be covered by risk-based population health and bundled-payment contracts.

- Sixty-three percent of leaders believe their hospital or health system will increase its participation in narrow insurance networks by 25 percent as a growth strategy.

Exhibit 1

Historical and Projected Federal Spending

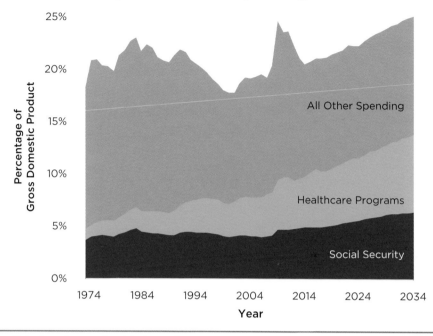

Source: Data from Congressional Budget Office.

—continued from pg. 5

(DRGs), which aimed to reduce unnecessary spending and increase awareness of the volume and efficacy of services provided (Porter and Teisberg 2006). The national implementation of DRGs signaled that the fee-for-service system was deeply flawed and fraught with fragmentation, siloed care, and a narrow rather than holistic view of patients' health. It also prevented providers from delivering meaningful, coordinated, and efficient care. If left unchecked, it would bring down America's healthcare system.

President George W. Bush furthered the transformation by tying payment reform to a population-level health focus. In 2006, by executive order, the Bush administration linked reimbursement to quality outcome measures, advanced the principles of price and quality transparency, promoted interoperable health information technology, and led early efforts to reward providers for value rather than volume. Those efforts were later accelerated by the passage of President Barack Obama's Affordable Care Act.

Today, multiple pathways exist to engage providers in the value movement and encourage them to accept more accountability and risk for patients' health and medical costs. One type of delivery and payment reform model,

the accountable care organization (ACO), has grown significantly over time (exhibit 2). In 2017, 923 ACOs covered 32 million lives—2.2 million more lives than in 2016 (Muhlestein, Saunders, and McClellan 2016).

The mandate for change is thus rooted in economics, and although politics will certainly have influence, it is unlikely to alter the shift to value-based care, which has already demonstrated promising results (McWilliams et al. 2015; Muhlestein, Saunders, and McClellan 2016). While the drivers of reform may oscillate between government payers, private payers, and state innovations, the overarching goal of lowering costs and improving quality will remain paramount.

Implications for Healthcare Leaders

Transcending the fog of the healthcare debate allows us to develop a new vision of healthcare's future and the economic imperatives that compel reform. It also helps us identify the abilities and critical success factors necessary to make the new vision a reality.

Overcoming barriers. Successfully moving to value-based care will require hospital and health system leaders to overcome barriers to change, especially the lack of readiness to manage

Exhibit 2

Growth of Accountable Care Organizations, 2011–2017: Estimated ACO Penetration by Hospital Referral Region

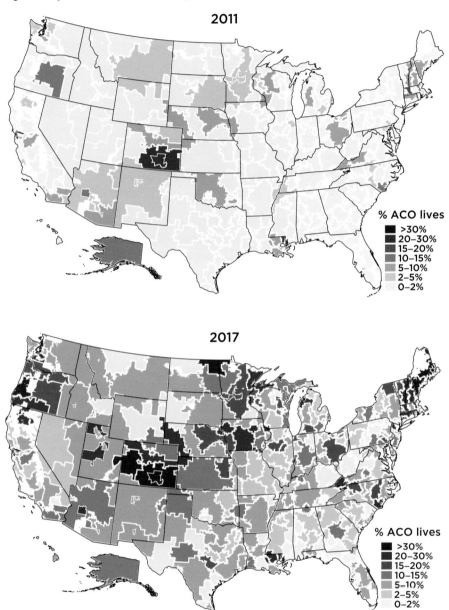

Source: Leavitt Partners ACO database.

patient populations in new and effective ways. Securing the buy-in of physicians, who are on the front lines of reimagining and reinventing patient care, is also critical.

Developing a common language.
Healthcare reform requires a common language. To enact meaningful change in the transition from fee-for-service to

value-based payment, we need to plant both feet in the world of value and keep pushing to create universal standards, definitions, and competencies. A common language does not mean a mandate from the government or a one-size-fits-all system that each state and community must enact. Rather, a common language must be developed through a collaboration of the private and public

spheres that provides clarity and guidance and embraces state and local flexibility. Standard definitions can align all stakeholders in healthcare toward the common goal of increased value, and multiple pathways should (and do) exist to reach that goal.

Transitioning to MACRA. The passage of MACRA (the Medicare Access and

CHIP Reauthorization Act) reflected bipartisan commitment to value-based reform and determination to spur more providers to begin (or advance) their transition to this model. MACRA incentivizes hospitals to look for opportunities to foster collaboration, increase coordination, and establish relationships with other healthcare organizations and payers.

Strategically, with MACRA's emphasis on alternative payment models (APMs), leaders should develop a pathway to move affiliated providers into advanced APMs. In the early stages of implementation, most hospitals will be subject to the Merit-Based Incentive Payment System (MIPS). However, MACRA rewards providers that progress along the risk spectrum by moving into advanced APMs, where they will receive a larger annual payment update, qualify for bonuses, and benefit from exemption from MIPS reporting.

Stabilizing Medicare. Today, Medicare covers nearly 60 million people and is expected to cover more than 81 million by 2030 (Moffit and Senger 2013). Maintaining the momentum of reforms, including Medicare ACOs and other value-based approaches, will be important. The Centers for Medicare & Medicaid Services (CMS) and the CMS Innovation Center have developed a variety of initiatives to achieve the Institute for Healthcare Improvement's Triple Aim of improving the patient experience, improving the health of populations, and lowering the cost of care (IHI 2017). The Trump administration may shift some of the responsibility for developing new payment and delivery systems from CMS to other groups, such as the Physician-Focused Payment Model Technical Advisory Committee (PTAC), but innovations must continue. CMS, PTAC, commercial payers, and other stakeholders can learn from the successes and failures of current and past efforts and design remedies that improve patient care, reduce spending, incentivize care coordination, and engage all types of providers.

Reengineering Medicaid. With more than 74 million beneficiaries,

Medicaid enrollment in the United States is bigger than the population of France (Medicaid.gov 2017). Congress is embroiled in debate over whether and how Medicaid expansion should be phased out or restructured entirely. Front-runner proposals for reengineering Medicaid include block grants and per capita spending with the ability to cap enrollment. Efforts to overhaul the program, however, must weigh the costs and consequences of potentially increasing the number of uninsured Americans.

As a low-income population often burdened with multiple chronic conditions, Medicaid patients present both challenges and opportunities to make meaningful reductions in spending and improvements in health. State Medicaid innovations can help guide healthcare's movement toward value. CMS Administrator Seema Verma has expressed her support for state-generated Medicaid solutions. Oregon's coordinated care organizations, for example, have shown promising reductions in spending and gains in quality by increasing their use of community health workers, social workers, and care coordinators (McConnell et al. 2017). Meanwhile, Indiana's Medicaid innovations stress increased patient engagement, responsibility, and cost sharing through health savings accounts (Verma and Neale 2016). Although the future of Medicaid is uncertain, in a capped-spending scenario, states clearly will be faced with the choice of either (1) reducing benefits and services and eliminating all nonessential expenses or (2) increasing efforts to maximize efficiency through payment and delivery system reform. Most states will do both, making them innovation laboratories worth watching.

Adopting new models of care. APMs aim to improve quality and lower cost by changing both physician reimbursement and care delivery. In ACOs, providers assume responsibility for the total cost of care for a defined population of patients, and they have more latitude to redesign care. For example, ACOs use teams of physicians and nonphysicians—including nurses, physical thera-

---

Transitioning to these new models of care takes time and requires the engagement of physicians, hospital executives, and policymakers.

---

pists, and social workers—to holistically address patients' needs, encourage preventive care, and help patients manage their chronic conditions. Under bundled payments, providers are responsible for the total cost of care for a specific episode. Whereas a fragmented fee-for-service system hampers high-value care, bundled payments incentivize physicians to more effectively collaborate across the care continuum. Transitioning to these new models of care, however, takes time and requires the engagement of physicians, hospital executives, and policymakers.

Collaborating for behavioral health. As healthcare becomes less siloed, leaders should develop collaborative affiliations with a variety of community groups that may include behavioral health clinics, schools, and social service agencies. Research shows that people with chronic conditions are more likely to have mental or substance abuse disorders and that those with behavioral health conditions often struggle with medication adherence and keeping regular appointments (Fraze et al. 2016). Hospitals will need to find ways to integrate physician and mental health care. The National Academy of Medicine's *Vital Directions for Health & Health Care* report calls for activating communities and jointly mobilizing resources (Dzau et al. 2017). Some ACOs have begun to address the nonmedical needs of patients that significantly impact their clinical health, including housing, food, and transportation. Effective alliances and partnerships between hospitals and local social service agencies may foster more meaningful improvements in population health.

Conclusion

Moving forward, healthcare executives must pursue the larger goals of transformation while developing customized strategies for the providers they currently work with. A variety of strategies are necessary to accommodate the diversity of provider specialties and patient needs. Driving the focus on value is recognition that fee-for-service creates the wrong incentives, that coordinated care is better than uncoordinated care, and that steps must be taken to control costs. Progress is being made, but not quickly enough. Innovative leaders who recognize the economic imperatives mandating change, coalesce around common standards and language, collaborate with other providers, and engage with alternative payment and delivery models will be rewarded.

References

Dzau, V.J., M. McClellan, S. Burke, M.J. Coye, T.A. Daschle, A. Diaz, W.H. Frist, M.E. Gaines, M.A. Hamburg, J.E. Henney, S. Kumanyika, M.O. Leavitt, J.M. McGinnis, R. Parker, L.G. Sandy, L.D. Schaeffer, G.D. Steele, P. Thompson, and E. Zerhouni. 2017. *Vital Directions for Health & Health Care: Priorities from a National Academy of Medicine Initiative*. National Academy of Medicine. Published March 21. https://nam.edu/vital-directions-for-health-health-care-priorities-from-a-national-academy-of-medicine-initiative/.

Fraze, T., V.A. Lewis, H.P. Rodriguez, and E.S. Fisher. 2016. "Housing, Transportation, and Food: How ACOs Seek to Improve Population Health by Addressing Nonmedical Needs of Patients." *Health Affairs* 35 (11): 2109–15.

Institute for Healthcare Improvement (IHI). 2017. "IHI Triple Aim Initiative." Accessed June 19. www.ihi.org/Engage/Initiatives/TripleAim/.

McConnell, K.J., S. Renfro, R.C. Lindrooth, D.J. Cohen, N.T. Wallace, and M.E. Chernew. 2017. "Oregon's Medicaid Reform and Transition to Global Budgets Were Associated with Reductions in Expenditures." *Health Affairs* 36 (3): 451–59.

McWilliams, J.M., M.E. Chernew, B.E. Landon, and A.L. Schwartz. 2015. "Performance Differences in Year 1 of Pioneer Accountable Care Organizations." *New England Journal of Medicine* 372 (20): 1927–36.

Medicaid.gov. 2017. "March 2017 Medicaid and CHIP Enrollment Data Highlights." Accessed June 19. www.medicaid.gov/medicaid/program-information/medicaid-and-chip-enrollment-data/report-highlights/.

Moffit, R., and A. Senger. 2013. "Medicare's Demographic Challenge—and the Urgent Need for Reform." The Heritage Foundation. Published March 21. www.heritage.org/health-care-reform/report/medicares-demographic-challenge-and-the-urgent-need-reform.

Muhlestein, D., R. Saunders, and M. McClellan. 2016. "Medicare Accountable Care Organization Results for 2015: The Journey to Better Quality and Lower Costs Continues." *Health Affairs Blog*. Published September 9. http://healthaffairs.org/blog/2016/09/09/medicare-accountable-care-organization-results-for-2015-the-journey-to-better-quality-and-lower-costs-continues/.

Porter, M.E., and E.O. Teisberg 2006. *Redefining Health Care: Creating Value-Based Competition on Results*. Boston: Harvard Business School Press.

Verma, S., and B. Neale. 2016. "Healthy Indiana 2.0 Is Challenging Medicaid Norms." *Health Affairs Blog*. Published August 29. http://healthaffairs.org/blog/2016/08/29/healthy-indiana-2-0-is-challenging-medicaid-norms/.

Consumerism in Healthcare: The Next Chapter

by Richard L. Gundling

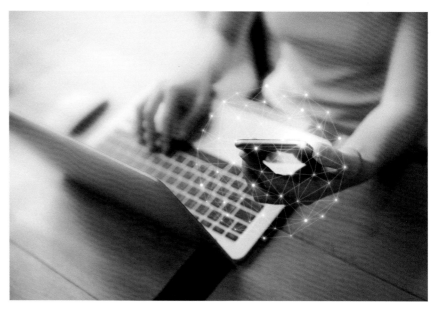

Healthcare consumers lived with uncertainty for much of 2017. As political battles were waged in Congress, both the future of the Affordable Care Act (ACA) and the specifics of prospective replacement legislation remained up in the air. Those who followed the news learned that legislation related to healthcare can affect people in all sectors of the insurance market, that the legislative process can be nontransparent and unpredictable, and that everything is fair game in politics.

In the wake of this experience, some consumers may feel that the health insurance guardrails are not as substantial as they seemed. Their anxiety about the stability of their insurance coverage and their ability to manage out-of-pocket expenses may be ratcheted up a notch, exacerbating their frustration with opaque healthcare pricing and fueling the demand for greater price transparency.

Apart from events in Washington, DC, consumerism is at an inflection point. The current generation of consumerism initiatives raised expectations—perhaps unrealistically so—and they have not always delivered. For example, high-deductible health plans, initially heralded as consumer driven, are now sometimes viewed as a blunt instrument that reduces both high-value and low-value utilization indiscriminately. Additionally, price transparency initiatives have not increased consumers' use of transparency tools or meaningfully supported their healthcare purchasing decisions. And providers are just beginning to embrace consumerism and to target financial interactions in their efforts to improve the patient experience. Against this backdrop, consumer concerns about price and affordability, amplified by social media, are threatening to erode the trust in hospitals and healthcare systems that once seemed unshakeable.

In the years ahead, physicians, hospitals, health systems, and health plans must collaborate with each other—and with consumers—to turn this ship around. In an encouraging sign, more than 90 percent of healthcare executives responding to the latest *Futurescan* national survey expect to develop or expand their formal processes for gaining insight into patients' preferences (e.g., through patient and family advisory councils) in the next five years.

About the Author

Richard L. Gundling, FHFMA, CMA, is senior vice president of healthcare financial practices at the Healthcare Financial Management Association (HFMA), where he is responsible for overseeing HFMA's technical and content direction; leading the organization's Washington, DC, activities; and managing its thought leadership efforts. Results from HFMA's policy initiatives have been used by hospitals, rating agencies, regulatory agencies, congressional committees, accounting standard–setting bodies, state hospital organizations, and other government and industry leaders. Gundling also serves as staff liaison to the HFMA Principles and Practices Board. He previously worked at the National Hospital for Orthopaedics and Rehabilitation, Prince William Hospital Corporation, and the Visiting Nurse Association of Northern Virginia. He is a fellow of HFMA, a certified management accountant, and a member of the Institute of Management Accountants. He has written extensively on healthcare finance and leadership topics.

FUTURESCAN SURVEY RESULTS
Consumerism

How likely is it that the following will happen by 2023?

Very Likely (%)	Somewhat Likely (%)	Neutral (%)	Somewhat Unlikely (%)	Very Unlikely (%)
31	38	21	8	3

Your hospital or health system will have implemented strategies to help ensure patients do not receive unexpected out-of-network bills associated with their care.

Very Likely (%)	Somewhat Likely (%)	Neutral (%)	Somewhat Unlikely (%)	Very Unlikely (%)
16	33	12	29	10

At least 50 percent of your hospital's or health system's patients will pay their medical bills using a mobile app on their smartphones.

Very Likely (%)	Somewhat Likely (%)	Neutral (%)	Somewhat Unlikely (%)	Very Unlikely (%)
19	37	15	24	6

More than 50 percent of your hospital's or health system's patients will review price and quality data with their physician before choosing where to receive care for "shoppable" healthcare services.

Very Likely (%)	Somewhat Likely (%)	Neutral (%)	Somewhat Unlikely (%)	Very Unlikely (%)
64	27	6	2	1

Your hospital or health system will develop or expand its formal processes for gaining insight into patients' preferences (e.g., patient and family advisory councils) to improve the patient experience.

Very Likely (%)	Somewhat Likely (%)	Neutral (%)	Somewhat Unlikely (%)	Very Unlikely (%)
54	29	14	3	◊

Your hospital or health system will have established a strategic goal to improve patient satisfaction scores related to the patient's financial experience.

Note: Percentages in each row may not sum exactly to 100% because of rounding.
◊ Less than 0.5%.

What Hospital Executives Anticipate by 2023

- Nearly two-thirds of respondents (64 percent) say it is very likely their organization will develop or expand efforts to gain insights into patient preferences.

- Eighty-three percent believe it is somewhat to very likely their hospital or health system will have a strategic goal to improve patients' satisfaction with their financial experience.

continued on pg. 13

—continued from pg. 11

Elevating the Financial Experience

As a previous *Futurescan* contributor noted, "the patient experience incorporates *every* facet of care provided in *every* setting, by *every* person, *every* day. Clinical expertise is no longer enough" (Dempsey 2016). Increasingly, healthcare leaders are realizing that a patient's financial experience is an important element of his or her overall healthcare encounter, one that affects not only patient satisfaction but also attitudes toward the hospital or system where the experience occurred. About 83 percent of *Futurescan* survey respondents believe it is somewhat to very likely that by 2023 their hospital or health system will establish a strategic goal to improve patient satisfaction scores related to the patient's financial experience. Clearly, there is work to be done: According to a recent study, one in four consumers in poor or fair health feels that their experience with hospital billing and payment has damaged their opinion of the organization (PwC Health Research Institute 2015).

Demystifying bills. Hospital bills have long been criticized for being difficult to understand. Efforts to make bills less confusing began in earnest with the Healthcare Financial Management Association's (HFMA's) Patient Friendly Billing® project in 2006 and are ongoing. In 2016, AARP collaborated with the US Department of Health & Human Services on a competition to redesign medical bills called "A Bill You Can Understand" (AARP 2017). In its design brief, RadNet, Inc. (one of the two winners) stated, "Empathy for the patient is the impetus behind our concept. Our main priority was to see billing through the eyes of the patient." This philosophy is informing the way forward-looking hospitals and health systems are approaching the entire financial experience.

Adopting best practices. The patient's financial experience begins with the first conversation about financial matters and concludes with resolution of the account. Although payment is no longer just a series of business-to-business transactions, hospital revenue cycle staff typically have little or no training to equip them for conversations with patients about sensitive financial matters. Furthermore, initiatives to improve quality by reducing process variability have yet to extend to the financial sphere. Foundational industry-consensus best practices developed in 2014 by a task force with representation from the American Hospital Association, America's Health Insurance Plans, and other healthcare stakeholders have been adopted by more than 240 hospitals as of late 2017; only low awareness of this free resource has limited widespread adoption (HFMA 2017).

Improving transparency. Healthcare consulting firm Oliver Wyman estimates that 40 to 70 percent of healthcare services can be considered "shoppable." Shoppability for certain services will increase in tandem with price transparency, according to Wyman, and shoppability "will influence hospitals' pricing across the board" (Bach 2017). Despite a flurry of activity in the price transparency arena in recent years, consumers still have trouble obtaining price and quality information for shoppable services in advance of receiving those services. Few use the price transparency tools that hospitals, health systems, health plans, and third-party organizations offer. One factor limiting the popularity of these tools is that they are harder to use than pricing tools in other sectors, such as airline travel. When comparing price information for an MRI becomes as easy as comparing airfares, assessments of consumers' propensity to shop for healthcare will be on more solid footing.

About 56 percent of *Futurescan* survey respondents believe it is somewhat to very likely

continued from pg. 12

- Sixty-nine percent of leaders consider it at least somewhat likely they will have implemented strategies to help ensure patients do not receive unexpected out-of-network bills for their care.

- Respondents are divided on whether patients will use mobile apps to pay their bills; 49 percent say this is somewhat to very likely, while 39 percent say it is somewhat to very unlikely.

that, in the next five years, more than half of their patients will review price and quality data with their physician before choosing where to receive care for shoppable services.

Preventing surprise bills. Surprise medical bills can arise when a patient receives care either at an in-network five years to help ensure patients do not receive unexpected out-of-network bills.

Paying the bill. Consumers who are accustomed to online shopping and household bill paying will expect hospital bill payment and out-of-pocket expense management to be integrated fire for failing to promote high-value healthcare.

The incorporation of preventive services in the ACA with no cost sharing is one example of benefit plan design that encourages high-value healthcare. Value-based insurance design, or V-BID, is another. V-BID seeks to reduce or remove financial barriers to essential, high-value clinical services. Patients' out-of-pocket costs (e.g., copayments) are aligned with the value of services in V-BID plans. For example, the copayment for a cardiologist visit after a heart attack is lower than the copayment for a dermatologist visit for mild acne.

Although V-BID is not new, it will receive a boost from the five-year Value-Based Insurance Design Model demonstration project launched by the Centers for Medicare & Medicaid Services (CMS) in 2017. The project allows Medicare Advantage plans in seven states to offer supplemental benefits or reduced cost sharing to enrollees with CMS-specified chronic conditions, focused on the services that are of highest clinical value to them (CMS 2017).

> Hospitals and health systems have the opportunity to use the payment process to differentiate themselves and build consumer trust, loyalty, and satisfaction.

facility from an out-of-network clinician or at an out-of-network facility. A medical bill for out-of-network care will be a surprise if the patient did not voluntarily choose the out-of-network clinician for care or was not aware that an out-of-network clinician or facility would be involved. A Connecticut study found that 60 percent of healthcare consumers do not realize that in-network hospitals can have out-of-network physicians (UConn Health Disparities Institute 2017). Another nationwide study conducted by researchers at the Federal Trade Commission found that in 2014, 20 percent of hospital inpatient admissions that originated in the emergency department (ED), 14 percent of outpatient visits to the ED, and 9 percent of elective inpatient admissions "likely led to a surprise medical bill" (Garmon and Chartock 2017).

Surprise bills have emerged as a source of financial anxiety and unanticipated medical debt for consumers. It is incumbent on hospitals, health systems, physicians, and health plans to take steps to inform patients about the risk of surprise bills and offer concrete information to help them avoid these unwelcome surprises. About 69 percent of respondents to the *Futurescan* survey think it is somewhat to very likely that their hospital or health system will implement strategies in the next and streamlined sooner rather than later. Today, there is an app to support virtually any purchase decision a consumer makes, whether it is parking a car downtown or buying a car. Likewise, consumers can do their banking and buy airline tickets on their phones. But although many hospitals offer online payment, only an estimated 3 to 4 percent currently have apps for this purpose. Nearly half of healthcare executives participating in the *Futurescan* survey say it is somewhat to very likely that by 2023 at least half of their patients will pay their medical bills using a mobile app on their smartphones.

Improving payment convenience can increase consumer loyalty. Hospitals and health systems have the opportunity to use the payment process to differentiate themselves and build consumer trust, loyalty, and satisfaction—just as airlines, restaurants, and retailers such as Amazon have done.

Designing Health Plans to Support Value

The quest for value in healthcare has focused on the provider sector. But providers understand that third-party support for high-value care will help them deliver such care. High-deductible health plans are the prevalent benefit plan design, and are likely to remain so, but they have increasingly come under

Implications for Healthcare Leaders

Implications for hospitals and health systems are straightforward, albeit not necessarily simple.

Build a solid foundation in financial interactions with patients. Hospital leaders should take a page from the clinical playbook by reducing unnecessary variation and standardizing their organization's approach to financial communications with patients. Revenue cycle and frontline staff will benefit from training to help them navigate financial conversations with patients effectively and empathetically. Efforts to deliver price and quality information that is accurate, timely, and easy to understand should be ramped up. Hospitals should inform patients about the risk of surprise medical bills, at a minimum, and consider steps they might take to reduce that risk. In uncertain times, consistency, clarity, empathy, and openness in financial interactions are particularly appreciated by consumers. Although modernizing payment systems through the development of apps and other technology-enabled tools will come to be expected, technology cannot replace a solid foundation in best practices.

Promote benefit designs that support value. Value-based payment incentivizes both hospitals and physicians to learn and practice high-value care. Health plans that take the long view will be motivated to incorporate V-BID principles and strategies into their existing benefit design and develop new V-BID products. Hospitals and health systems should consider engaging in conversations with their health plans and exploring the feasibility of partnering with them on V-BID pilots that reflect the health status and health challenges of their respective patient populations. Provider-owned health plans and self-insured hospitals and health systems may be well positioned to fast-track these pilot projects.

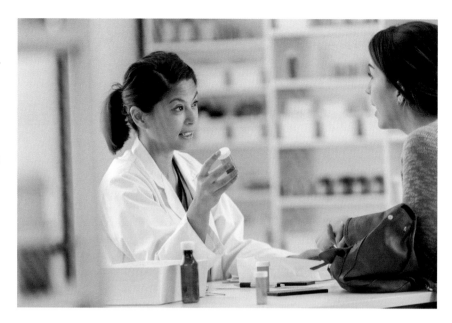

Conclusion

The quest for value is the common thread uniting consumerism initiatives by various stakeholders, including hospitals, health systems, physicians, and health plans. Although stakeholders have traditionally had conflicting interests, the time for finger-pointing and kicking the can down the road is over. As the volume-to-value transformation picks up steam, healthcare stakeholders must collaborate to deliver improved value to the people they serve. Value is the essence of consumerism.

References

AARP. 2017. "'A Bill You Can Understand' Design & Innovation Challenge." Accessed August 26. www.abillyoucan understand.com.

Bach, B. 2017. "Shoppable Healthcare Services and Future Pricing." Oliver Wyman Health. Published May 18. http://health.oliverwyman.com/transform-care/2017/05/infographic_shoppab.html.

Centers for Medicare & Medicaid Services (CMS). 2017. "Medicare Advantage Value-Based Insurance Design Model." Updated August 17. https://innovation.cms.gov/initiatives/vbid.

Dempsey, C. 2016. "The Evolution of the Patient Experience." In *Futurescan 2016–2021: Healthcare Trends and Implications*, 6–10. Chicago: Society for Healthcare Strategy & Market Development of the American Hospital Association and the American College of Healthcare Executives.

Garmon, C., and B. Chartock. 2017. "One in Five Inpatient Emergency Department Cases May Lead to Surprise Bills." *Health Affairs* 36 (1): 177–81.

Healthcare Financial Management Association (HFMA). 2017. *Patient Financial Communications Best Practices*. Accessed August 26. www.hfma.org/WorkArea/DownloadAsset.aspx?id=19968.

PwC Health Research Institute. 2015. *Money Matters: Billing and Payment for a New Health Economy*. Published May. www.pwc.com/us/en/health-industries/health-research-institute/publications/pdf/pwc-hri-healthcare-billing-and-payments.pdf.

UConn Health Disparities Institute. 2017. *Measuring Health Insurance Literacy in Connecticut*. Published April. https://health.uconn.edu/health-disparities/wp-content/uploads/sites/53/2017/04/HIL-Brief-4_2017.pdf.

Healthcare's Moment of Cyber Reckoning

by John Riggi and Patrick Pilch

If WannaCry taught us anything, it's that health-care has its own kidnapping-for-ransom problem. Only it's not people being held hostage—it's their data.

The May 2017 WannaCry ransomware attack hit healthcare hardest, incapacitating 47 of the United Kingdom's 248 National Health System trusts, some of which took days to recover. Although hospitals in the United States came away from WannaCry relatively unscathed, their leaders aren't exactly confident in their defenses against future cyber attacks. About 83 percent of hospital CEOs and other leaders who participated in this year's *Futurescan* national survey believe it is at least somewhat likely that a hospital or health system in their service area will experience a cyber attack in the next five years involving the theft of patient data from a cloud services provider. In fact, around the time the survey was conducted, a ransom-ware attack on an Arkansas provider breached the data of almost 130,000 patients, locking the organization out of its files, medical images, and patient visit information (Davis 2017).

The number of data breaches in the United States has been increasing steadily since 2010 (exhibit 1), and they have also become more diverse and severe (exhibit 2). Through the third quarter of 2017, healthcare organizations in the United States had reported 210 large-scale data breaches, defined by the US Department of Health & Human Services (HHS) as those affecting 500 or more individuals. Of the entities that reported breaches, 82 percent were providers, so more than 2.6 million individuals were collectively affected. Hacking and ransom-ware attacks were behind 41 percent of the breaches (OCR 2017).

Healthcare leaders are showing profound concern, and rightfully so. About 51 percent of those responding to the *Futurescan* survey predict that, in the next five years, they will see a cybersecurity breach in their service area that interferes with critical medical systems and causes harm to at least one patient.

It's no secret that hackers have been homing in on healthcare as a target for a while. The WannaCry attack simply highlighted the field's vulnerabilities.

But what makes healthcare so vulnerable to cyber threats?

First, it is the only industry charged with handling valuable bulk data sets that combine personal health information (PHI), personally identifiable information, payment information, medical research, and intellectual property—making healthcare especially lucrative for cyber criminals and nation-states.

Second, a combination of factors—a lack of resources devoted specifically to cybersecurity, the complexity of health networks, and a vast array of internet-connected devices—leaves healthcare open to risks from multiple attack vectors.

Finally, many hospitals and health systems still rely on older technologies, perhaps because they prioritize immediate access to data over data security.

About the Authors

John Riggi leads BDO's cybersecurity and financial crimes practice. He is a highly decorated veteran of the Federal Bureau of Investigation (FBI), where he spent nearly 30 years. In the FBI's cyber division, he led the national program to develop mission-critical partnerships with healthcare and other infrastructure industries, which was essential to the investigation and exchange of information related to national security and criminal cyber threats.

Patrick Pilch is the national coleader of The BDO Center for Healthcare Excellence & Innovation. He has more than 30 years of experience in healthcare, financial services, operational management, and restructuring. Pilch works with BDO's clinical and business advisory professionals to help healthcare organizations thrive in an era of daunting challenge and boundless opportunity.

Cybersecurity

How likely is it that the following will happen by 2023?

Very Likely (%)	Somewhat Likely (%)	Neutral (%)	Somewhat Unlikely (%)	Very Unlikely (%)
42	41	14	3	1

A hospital or health system in your service area will have experienced a cybersecurity attack involving the theft of patient data from a cloud services provider.

| 72 | 23 | 5 | 0 | ◊ |

Your hospital or health system will increase its investment in advanced cybersecurity defense technology capable of detecting and preventing attacks without human intervention.

| 16 | 35 | 35 | 12 | 2 |

A hospital or health system in your service area will have experienced a cybersecurity breach that interferes with critical medical systems and causes physical harm to one or more patients.

| 45 | 36 | 17 | 1 | 1 |

Your hospital or health system will have purchased additional insurance to protect against the potential costs associated with a cybersecurity attack (e.g., care interruption, civil liability, regulatory exposure, incident response or recovery).

| 26 | 44 | 21 | 8 | 1 |

Because of the increased threat of attacks and breaches, your hospital or health system will have outsourced at least some of its cybersecurity functions to a specialized management services provider.

Note: Percentages in each row may not sum exactly to 100% because of rounding.
◊ Less than 0.5%.

What Hospital Executives Anticipate by 2023

- Seven in ten respondents (72 percent) think it is very likely they will increase investment in advanced cybersecurity defense technology.

- Eighty-three percent believe it is at least somewhat likely a hospital or health system in their area will experience a cyber attack.

- Eighty-one percent of leaders say it is somewhat to very likely their organization will purchase additional insurance to protect against a data breach.

- Nearly three-quarters (70 percent) believe it is somewhat to very likely their hospital or health system will outsource some of its cybersecurity functions.

Exhibit 1

Number of Large-Scale Breaches by Year

2010	2011	2012	2013	2014	2015	2016
199	200	218	277	312	269	327

Source: OCR (2017).
Note: Individual reports of a breach may involve one or more types of breach (e.g., theft, loss). As a result, the number of reported incidents or breaches in a specific year may reflect double counting.

Exhibit 2

Top Ten Large-Scale US Healthcare Data Breaches (Through Third Quarter 2017)

Location	Patients Affected	Date Submitted to Office of Civil Rights	Breach Type	Location of Breached Information
Kentucky	697,800	March 1, 2017	Theft	Other
Michigan	500,000	June 16, 2017	Hacking/IT incident (ransomware)	Network server
Texas	279,663	March 22, 2017	Hacking/IT incident (ransomware)	Network server
California	266,123	August 10, 2017	Hacking/IT incident	Network server
Arkansas	128,000	September 24, 2017	Hacking/IT incident	Network server
Michigan	106,008	August 24, 2017	Hacking/IT incident	Network server
Pennsylvania	93,323	April 28, 2017	Hacking/IT incident	Network server
Indiana	85,995	March 2, 2017	Hacking/IT incident	Network server
Missouri	80,270	March 25, 2017	Hacking/IT incident	E-mail
Georgia	79,930	February 21, 2017	Hacking/IT incident	Other

Source: OCR (2017).
Note: IT = information technology.

continued from pg. 16

The *Futurescan* survey shows healthcare leaders are willing to ramp up their cyber protections. About 72 percent indicated that, by 2023, they are very likely to increase their investment in advanced cybersecurity defense technology capable of detecting and preventing attacks without human intervention. About 23 percent, meanwhile, said they are somewhat likely to do so, and almost none said they are unlikely to do so.

Playing Catch-Up

While other industries, such as financial services, have been quicker to modify their security controls to keep pace with the digital transformation, healthcare has often lagged behind.

But as regulators such as HHS's Office for Civil Rights (OCR), the Food and Drug Administration (FDA), and the Department of Justice (DOJ) heighten their scrutiny—and enforcement actions—around cybersecurity, providers will need to modernize their security controls or face the consequences.

OCR scrutiny. Underscoring the increased financial liabilities at stake when it comes to cybersecurity regulation by the OCR, one Midwest provider reached a record $5.55 million settlement with the agency in August 2016 for violations of the Health Insurance Portability and Accountability Act (HIPAA). The violations involved breached electronic PHI for more than 4 million individuals. The organization agreed to pay the settlement and adopt a corrective action plan (HHS 2016).

At the same time, the OCR announced its intention to more widely investigate breaches affecting fewer than 500 individuals through its regional offices (HIPAA Journal 2016).

In 2017, the OCR began conducting on-site audits of hospitals to ensure that policies and procedures are in place to address privacy rule controls, breach notification rule controls, and security risk controls. HIPAA-covered entities have ten days to respond to an OCR audit (Sullivan 2016).

FDA scrutiny. The increased security scrutiny that device manufacturers and their provider partners face was demonstrated in 2017 when the FDA notified the public of cybersecurity vulnerabilities relating to implantable cardiac devices from St. Jude Medical (FDA 2017).

The notification came after a St. Jude investor made accusations that the company's pacemakers and defibrillators were vulnerable to cyber attack. Stock prices declined as a result, and reputations were damaged.

The news surfaced a year after the FDA released guidance on postmarket cybersecurity vulnerabilities for medical devices, deeming manufacturers responsible for notifying the agency in the event they have to address issues that could pose a health risk (FDA 2016).

The guidance outlined several important postmarket actions:

- Monitoring cybersecurity information sources for identification of vulnerabilities and risks
- Detecting and assessing the presence and impact of a vulnerability
- Establishing and communicating protocols to address vulnerabilities
- Defining essential clinical performance to develop controls that protect, respond to, and recover from cybersecurity risk
- Adopting a multidisciplinary vulnerability disclosure policy and practice
- Deploying controls that address cybersecurity threats before a vulnerability can be exploited

"This guidance . . . emphasizes that manufacturers should monitor, identify, and address cybersecurity vulnerabilities . . . as part of their postmarket management of medical devices," the FDA stated. "[It] establishes a risk-based framework for assessing when changes to medical devices for cybersecurity

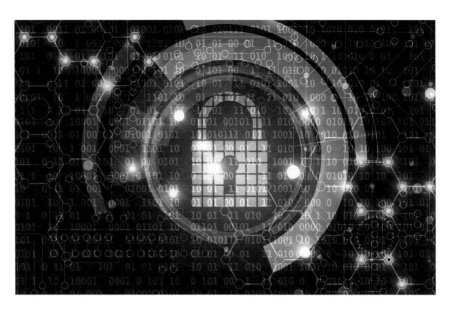

vulnerabilities require reporting to the agency" (FDA 2016).

DOJ scrutiny. Even as the OCR and FDA are increasing efforts to mitigate cybersecurity risks—and enforce compliance with industry security guidelines—the DOJ is ramping up its criminal enforcement actions against healthcare fraud. Because of a June 2016 Supreme Court decision, noncompliance with cybersecurity standards could fall under the purview of such enforcement actions.

Most recently, in July 2017, the DOJ announced the largest-ever healthcare fraud enforcement action by the Medicare Fraud Strike Force—involving 412 charged defendants across 41 federal districts, among them 115 doctors, nurses, and other licensed medical professionals—for their alleged participation in fraud schemes totaling $1.3 billion in false billings (DOJ 2017).

The move followed a June 2016 enforcement action alleging that 301 clinical professionals submitted $900 million in false Medicare claims (DOJ 2016) and the June 2016 Supreme Court decision that widened the net for whistle-blowers under the False Claims Act (FCA) (Pilch et al. 2016).

The Supreme Court decision, *Universal Health Services, Inc. v. United States ex rel. Escobar*, upheld the "implied false certification" theory of liability of the FCA, which aims to both prevent defrauding the government and penalize

those who commit such fraud. The theory treats a Medicaid payment request as an "implied certification of compliance" with pertinent statutes, regulations, or contract requirements—including those related to cybersecurity—material to conditions of payment. Notably, the Supreme Court decision clarified *material* broadly as "having a natural tendency to influence, or be capable of influencing, the payment or receipt of money or property."

The ruling came on the heels of the beginning of the transition to value-based reimbursement—thus at a time when healthcare costs were coming under greater scrutiny.

Takeaways

Providers are being held to greater levels of accountability not only for their own compliance with regulators' evolving cybersecurity guidance but also for that of their partners in the care continuum. And as their reimbursements are increasingly being tied to care quality rather than quantity, the Supreme Court decision creates the potential for greater risk under the FCA as it relates to security.

What matters most is not how a state or federal government labels relevant laws or requirements for payment, but whether defendants knowingly violate a condition they know to be "material" to a Medicaid payment decision. Under the cybersecurity lens, if an organization bills for services rendered but the quality of those services does not comply with security requirements—or if the organization is aware of a potential vulnerability but fails to disclose it—the organization could be deemed noncompliant with the FCA.

> Hospital and health system executives should develop a cybersecurity strategy and foster a corporate culture that solidifies proper defense and postmortem measures.

For an FDA-regulated medical device manufacturer, consequences could also include a costly device recall and having to resubmit the device for FDA approval.

Mitigating Risk and Improving Cyber Defenses

Because cybersecurity risks will only continue to grow in healthcare, hospital and health system executives should develop a cybersecurity strategy and foster a corporate culture that solidifies proper defense and postmortem measures. In working to create a well-designed cybersecurity program, organizations should do the following:

- **Remember the human element.** Change user behavior by introducing a training program based on employees' organizational roles and by implementing best practices for cyber hygiene.

- **Implement a risk-based, threat-driven patch management program.** Organizations should be able to identify system vulnerabilities and implement patches quickly. One way to do this is to outsource at least some cybersecurity functions to a specialized management services provider. According to the *Futurescan* survey, about 70 percent of healthcare leaders say they are at least somewhat likely to take this step in the next five years because of the increased threat of attacks and breaches.

- **Monitor continuously.** Organizations need threat monitoring and analytics tools to detect an attack, as well as investigative and digital forensic capabilities to understand what went wrong and assess the damage.

- **Develop a crisis communications plan.** This plan should include both internal and external communications and be aligned with an existing enterprise risk management framework.

- **Implement cybersecurity insurance claims preparedness and ensure that coverage is adequate.** Identify and quantify incurred event response costs for inclusion in an insurance claim. The *Futurescan* survey indicates that about 81 percent of healthcare leaders are at least somewhat likely to purchase additional insurance by 2023 to protect their organization against the potential costs associated with a cybersecurity attack.

For healthcare, a cyber attack—especially a ransomware infection that blocks access to critical medical data—is a human safety issue. Responding quickly can be a matter of life or death.

Providers have to make sure their defense measures keep pace with their technological advances—or else face the growing consequences.

References

Davis, J. 2017. "Ransomware Attack Breaches 128,000 Patient Records at Arkansas Provider." *Healthcare IT News*. Published October 2. www.healthcareitnews.com/news/ransomware-attack-breaches-128000-patient-records-arkansas-provider.

HIPAA Journal. 2016. "OCR to Increase Investigations of Small PHI Breaches." Published August 18. www.hipaajournal.com/ocr-to-increase-investigations-of-small-phi-breaches-3558/.

Pilch, P., G. Pomerantz, S. Giammarco, and D. Ventricelli. 2016. "Could Supreme Court Ruling on the False Claims Act Provide Whistleblowers a Wider Net?" BDO. Published July. www.bdo.com/insights/industries/healthcare/bdo-knows-healthcare-alert-july-2016.

Sullivan, T. 2016. "OCR: Onsite HIPAA Audits Coming in 2017." *Healthcare IT News*. Published December 7. www.healthcareitnews.com/news/ocr-onsite-hipaa-audits-coming-2017.

US Department of Health & Human Services (HHS). 2016. "Resolution Agreement and Corrective Action Plan Between OCR and Advocate Health Care Network." Published August 4. www.hhs.gov/sites/default/files/Advocate_racap.pdf.

US Department of Health & Human Services Office for Civil Rights (OCR). 2017. "Breach Portal: Notice to the Secretary of HHS Breach of Unsecured Protected Health Information." Accessed July 14. https://ocrportal.hhs.gov/ocr/breach/breach_report.jsf.

US Department of Justice (DOJ). 2017. "National Health Care Fraud Takedown Results in Charges Against over 412 Individuals Responsible for $1.3 Billion in Fraud Losses." Published July 13. www.justice.gov/opa/pr/national-health-care-fraud-takedown-results-charges-against-over-412-individuals-responsible.

———. 2016. "June 2016 Takedown." Published June 22. www.justice.gov/criminal-fraud/health-care-fraud-unit/june-2015-takedown.

US Food and Drug Administration (FDA). 2017. "Cybersecurity Vulnerabilities Identified in St. Jude Medical's Implantable Cardiac Devices and Merlin@home Transmitter: FDA Safety Communication." Published January 9. www.fda.gov/MedicalDevices/Safety/AlertsandNotices/ucm535843.htm.

———. 2016. "Postmarket Management of Cybersecurity in Medical Devices: Guidance for Industry and Food and Drug Administration Staff." Published December 28. www.fda.gov/downloads/medicaldevices/deviceregulationandguidance/guidancedocuments/ucm482022.pdf.

Dismantling Disparities: How Hospitals and Health Systems Can Advance Health Equity

by Eugene A. Woods, FACHE

If an outcome is seen to a greater or lesser extent between populations, there is disparity. And unfortunately, disparities in health are a persistent and well-documented problem plaguing our communities. As healthcare leaders, we likely feel a great responsibility when it comes to this topic because disparities in health could be directly influenced by disparities in the health*care* that we provide to different groups.

Of course, another significant force is contributing to these health disparities: namely, the social contexts in which people live, learn, work, play, and worship. Social determinants of health—factors such as education; exposure to discrimination; and access to safe housing, healthy food, transportation, and job opportunities—have a major effect on a person's health and quality of life (HHS 2017b).

This reality in no way minimizes the role that healthcare plays in the disparities problem. Indeed, healthcare disparities—differences across groups in health insurance coverage, access to care, and quality of care—function together with social determinants of health as dual factors in a complex and devastating equation.

But by working to counteract these joint forces, we can move the needle toward health equity: attainment of the highest level of health for all people (HHS 2017a). Health equity is achieved through intentional efforts to reduce healthcare disparities and positively influence health's social determinants. In short, it is social justice in health.

What's the Impact of Health Disparities?

The human toll of health disparities is enormous. Consider the following:

- Native American adults have a higher incidence of diabetes than does any other race or ethnicity in the United States (CDC 2017).
- African American babies are more than twice as likely as white babies to die before their first birthday (Mathews, MacDorman, and Thomas 2015).
- Under the scourge of our nation's current opioid epidemic, heroin use among white males has surged higher than in any other group (Madras 2017).

The impact is equally real on an economic level. Racial health disparities alone account for an estimated $35 billion in extra healthcare expenditures each year and $10 billion in lost productivity due to illness (LaVeist, Gaskin, and Richard 2011).

About the Author

Eugene A. (Gene) Woods is one of today's most prominent leaders in healthcare. He is president and CEO of Carolinas Health-Care System, one of the largest integrated health systems in the nation, with approximately 65,000 teammates at more than 900 care locations in North Carolina, South Carolina, and Georgia. Woods also served as 2017 chairman of the board of trustees of the American Hospital Association. Over a wide-ranging career spanning more than 25 years, Woods has guided not-for-profit and for-profit hospitals, academic and community-based delivery systems, and rural and urban facilities. Before joining Carolinas HealthCare System in April 2016, he was president and chief operating officer of CHRISTUS Health, based in Irving, Texas. Prior to that, he served as CEO of Saint Joseph Health System in Lexington, Kentucky, and chief operating officer of the Washington Hospital Center in Washington, DC. Woods holds master's degrees in business administration and health administration from Pennsylvania State University.

FUTURESCAN SURVEY RESULTS
Equity of Care

How likely is it that the following will happen by 2023?

Very Likely (%)	Somewhat Likely (%)	Neutral (%)	Somewhat Unlikely (%)	Very Unlikely (%)
40	39	11	10	◊

The racial and ethnic demographics of your hospital's or health system's workforce will mirror the demographics of the communities you serve.

57	33	7	3	1

At least 90 percent of your hospital's or health system's patients will have accurate data about their race, ethnicity, and preferred language recorded in their electronic medical records.

58	29	9	3	◊

Your hospital or health system will have provided cultural competency education to caregivers and other staff who interact with patients at the bedside.

48	36	11	5	0

Your hospital or health system will have implemented standardized collection of data regarding social determinants of health (e.g., economic, employment, education, housing, transportation) for the communities it serves.

52	32	12	3	2

Your hospital or health system will have incorporated health equity into its strategic plan, with an emphasis on quality and patient experience metrics.

66	25	6	3	0

Your hospital or health system will have used a data-driven process to identify high utilizers of healthcare in a defined region to guide targeted interventions that address patient needs, improve the quality of care, or reduce costs.

Note: Percentages in each row may not sum exactly to 100% because of rounding.
◊ Less than 0.5%.

What Hospital Executives Anticipate by 2023

- Two-thirds of respondents (66 percent) believe it is very likely their hospital or health system will use a data-driven process to identify high utilizers of services to deliver targeted healthcare.

continued on pg. 24

—continued from pg. 22

Clearly, health disparities are a serious problem. But before healthcare leaders can really work on influencing healthcare's role in the equation, we need to understand what led us here in the first place.

How Did We Get Here?

For a long time, hospitals weren't exactly encouraged or rewarded to keep people healthy. Fee-for-service models incen-

What Trends Are We Seeing?

Hospital and health system leaders know that health equity must be made a priority, and fortunately the number of available tools to do this is growing. Following are the latest trends driving advances in health equity.

Big data. The collection, analysis, and use of information to enact and measure effective change are among the

and ethnic stratification to predictive analytics, big data is here to stay.

Workforce optimization. More and more healthcare leaders are realizing that, to best serve the needs of diverse patient populations, our workforce must better reflect those populations. Only then can we ensure that the cultures and preferences of our patients are being considered and incorporated into how we provide care.

> Hospital and health system leaders know that health equity must be made a priority, and fortunately the number of available tools to do this is growing.

tivized just that: a higher quantity of services. As a result, true indicators of patient health, such as lower incidence of disease and fewer readmissions, were considered less important—and often worked directly against the hospital's bottom line.

Fortunately, healthcare is undergoing a significant transformation. As hospitals shift from a volume-based model to a value-based one, patients are deriving more real benefit from their care—both in dollar terms and in impact on their health and wellness.

The shift is valuable for the field, too, because it results in better coordination of care services and greater efficiencies across the care spectrum.

most potent and underused weapons at our disposal today—and the importance of big data will only continue to grow.

A particularly useful and promising data-driven process is hotspotting, a method for identifying patterns and outcomes in a specific region or group. Through visualization of data sets at the neighborhood or zip-code level, previously hidden relationships between geography and health outcomes become visible (AHA 2016). Ultimately, this insight offers the opportunity to plan and enact more targeted approaches to affecting a population's health.

Hotspotting is just one of many data collection methods. From patient racial

Training our staff is also key. Are they being educated on culturally competent care and equipped to have cross-cultural conversations with patients? Are they encouraged to cultivate a workplace environment in which different cultures and groups are acknowledged, embraced, and celebrated? It's much easier to foster an atmosphere of inclusivity for patients when we're walking the walk ourselves.

Collaboration 2.0. Working together with community partners isn't new, but the scope of these relationships is broadening, and the level of collaboration among seemingly unlikely community players is increasing.

From health systems, foundations, and nonprofits to insurance companies and even private businesses, partnerships are forming among a wide range of disparate groups—including some outside of healthcare. By pooling our knowledge and pulling our collective weight, we're tackling the multifaceted problem of health disparities from all angles.

The more we work together, the farther we can go in our calling to serve others. To keep our progress moving

continued from pg. 23

- Nine in ten leaders (90 percent) say it is somewhat to very likely that at least 90 percent of their patients will have accurate information about their race and other factors recorded in their electronic medical records.

- Eighty-seven percent think it is at least somewhat likely they will provide training in cultural competencies to staff who have bedside contact with patients.

- More than half of respondents (52 percent) say it is very likely their organization will incorporate health equity into its strategic plan. Another 32 percent believe it is somewhat likely.

forward, the American Hospital Association (AHA) launched the #123forEquity Campaign to Eliminate Health Care Disparities in 2015. As immediate past chairman of the AHA board of trustees, I personally encourage all AHA member hospitals to take the pledge and commit to delivering equitable care to all the patients they serve. (Visit www.equityof care.org for more information.) Taking the pledge and committing to its efforts are a fantastic first step in propelling your organization toward greater health equity.

How Hospitals Can Lead the Way

As a hospital or health system leader, how can you help move the needle in advancing health equity?

First, incorporate health equity goals and outcome measures into your organization's strategic plan. Doing so not only provides a framework and direction for your health equity work—it also sends a clear message that you have made the effort a priority.

You can also lead the way in advancing health equity in the following practical ways, both within and outside your hospital's walls.

Enhance your workforce's cultural competency. Your frontline staff are the face, hands, and heart of your hospital, so equip them with the skills they need to communicate with and care for diverse populations.

Only recently have we begun to embrace the nuanced and radical diversity of our nation's population and to focus on building true cross-cultural skills. This could mean training providers to ask thoughtful questions that create a dialogue with patients about their health, equipping providers with enhanced motivational interviewing skills, or educating them on working more collaboratively with interpreters. Such cross-cultural skills create the deep, authentic level of engagement with patients that makes us true partners in their health.

Collect relevant patient data. If your health system hasn't done so already, begin to capture REAL (race, ethnicity,

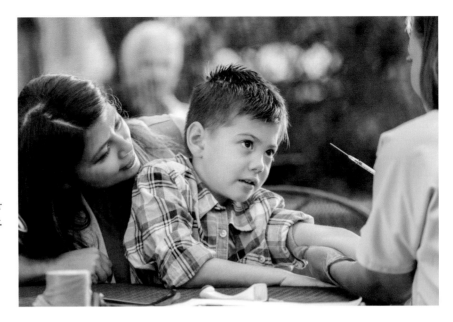

and language) data for your patients. Increasingly, SOGI (sexual orientation and gender identity) data are being collected as well. Collecting these data is the first goal of the AHA's Equity of Care pledge, and it's a great place to start in meeting the health equity challenge.

Looking at REAL and SOGI data helps your hospital see your community in a more nuanced way that goes beyond simple geographic or payer-mix distinctions, so you don't miss patterns of care that need to be addressed or overlook issues that are springing up in the communities you serve.

Having a standardized way to collect these data is critical. (A good place to start is the AHA Health Research & Educational Trust's Disparities Toolkit.) Patients should also be given the opportunity to identify themselves rather than be identified by hospital staff members.

Ideally, the data you collect will grow to include a more granular set of ethnicities, languages, and other characteristics over time, allowing you to get to know your patient population on a deeper level.

Review and analyze the data effectively. To ensure your efforts are worthwhile, establish a regular cadence for reviewing the data you gather. Ideally, a team of both administrators and clinicians is involved in this review. A fruitful way to view the information you've collected is to overlay REAL data on top of reports you

already generate, such as reports for clinical quality and patient experience metrics.

Next, cascade the relevant data to the frontline staff who are best poised to act on the information. For example, if a provider receives a report detailing all recent A1c and body mass index screenings he has performed, with the data presented and stratified by race and ethnicity, he can see which of his patients might be receiving inequitable care—and much more quickly than before.

At Carolinas HealthCare System, we're developing a similar process so that we can change course when the data show a concerning trend. For example, when one of our family practice locations viewed its colon cancer screening rates stratified by race and ethnicity, it found a lower screening rate in its Hispanic population. The practice created a Spanish-language video about the benefits of colon cancer screening for patients to view while waiting to see their doctor. Ultimately, the rate of colon cancer screening among the practice's Hispanic patients increased by more than 40 percent.

Use data to learn about your community. Look at data sources both inside and outside your hospital to determine where and why people are slipping through the cracks in your community.

More specifically, analyze factors such as access to care and high rates of emergency department utilization. Collect data from your patients on their social determinants of health. Review data from community health needs assessments and other outside sources. Implement geographic hotspotting to get a clearer picture of how the behaviors or outcomes of different groups are being affected.

At Carolinas HealthCare System, hotspotting has shown us where access to primary care is lacking in the Charlotte community. We've responded by opening new clinics, exploring the use of mobile care, and partnering with the YMCA of Greater Charlotte to embed care providers in its locations.

Collaborate with community partners to address broader issues. Hospitals and health systems often wield substantial political weight in their communities. It's time we started leveraging this influence to address broader issues that directly and indirectly affect our communities' health. There are numerous social determinants of health that we can influence by partnering with others, including public transportation, food deserts, school nutrition, patterns of violence, and lack of economic opportunities.

The opportunity for community collaboration around these issues is vast. For example, at Carolinas HealthCare System, we recently established an alliance with Bank of America and Novant Health, our region's other major health system, to form ONE Charlotte, an initiative that aims to remove barriers to employment and healthcare in our city.

Make your voice heard in larger policy conversations. The same influence you bring to community collaborations can be leveraged with local and state legislatures to enact lasting policy change. By getting involved, you can use your voice to better inform policy makers about the positive or negative consequences that emerging laws and funding decisions can have on your community's health—even when those laws and funding choices appear, on the surface, to have nothing to do with health.

It's Worth the Effort

Much work has yet to be done in reducing the prevalence of health disparities and achieving health equity. We must use every tool at our disposal and strive to influence every factor within our control. One great way to get started is to take the AHA's Equity of Care pledge.

We must use data to see our communities more clearly, to recognize disparities in the care we deliver, and to change course when we see a problem emerging or worsening. We must ensure our workforce understands, respects, and actually looks like the communities we serve. And we must collaborate with partners, both obvious and unexpected, to bring about necessary change outside our walls.

It's hard work. But a look at the patients and communities we serve shows it's well worth the effort. After all, population health is really just the collective health of individuals—of real people with real lives that have immense value.

A future where individuals have the chance to reach their highest potential for health regardless of where they live, what language they speak, or what they look like: That is the promising vision within our reach. With the right road map, and a firm resolve, we can make it happen.

References

American Hospital Association (AHA). 2016. *Next Generation of Community Health*. Accessed September 15, 2017. www.aha.org/content/17/committee-on-research-next-gen-community-health.pdf.

Centers for Disease Control and Prevention (CDC). 2017. "Native Americans with Diabetes." Published January. www.cdc.gov/vitalsigns/aian-diabetes/index.html.

LaVeist, T.A., D. Gaskin, and P. Richard. 2011. "Estimating the Economic Burden of Racial Health Inequalities in the United States." *International Journal of Health Services* 41 (2): 231–38.

Madras, B.K. 2017. "The Surge of Opioid Use, Addiction, and Overdoses." *JAMA Psychiatry* 74 (5): 441–42.

Mathews, T.J., M.F. MacDorman, and M.E. Thomas. 2015. "Infant Mortality Statistics from the 2013 Period Linked Birth/Infant Death Data Set." *National Vital Statistics Reports* 64 (9): 1–30.

US Department of Health & Human Services (HHS). 2017a. "Disparities." Healthy People 2020. Accessed July 13. www.healthypeople.gov/2020/about/foundation-health-measures/Disparities.

———. 2017b. "Social Determinants of Health." Healthy People 2020. Accessed June 28. www.healthypeople.gov/2020/topics-objectives/topic/social-determinants-of-health.

The Transformation of Emergency Care in the United States

by James J. Augustine, MD

Perhaps nowhere is the transformation of healthcare happening faster and more dramatically than in emergency medicine. In this volatile environment, where is the field headed? How should hospitals and health systems respond to remain competitive and best serve their communities in the future?

The answers to these multifaceted questions are being shaped by the convergence of a number of market forces.

Changing Consumer Expectations

Consumers are increasingly demanding emergency care when and how they want it. Ever more sensitive to cost and value, patients are playing a more proactive role in choosing how their healthcare dollar is spent. Just as important, patients' service and quality expectations, shaped by their transactions with other industries, are influencing their behavior. Anytime/anywhere availability, up-front price transparency, and an intentionally designed consumer experience are hallmarks of successful companies in the banking and retail sectors, for instance. Patients now expect the same from healthcare.

Pressure on Medical Costs

All types of insurers and businesses are endeavoring to lower healthcare costs by

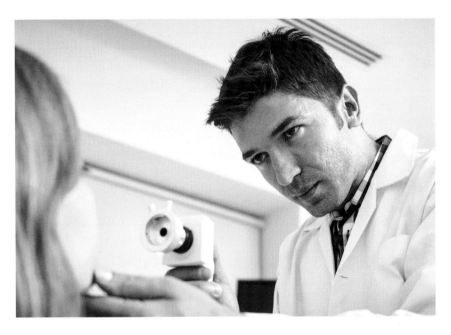

tightening reimbursement and requiring patients to make their own decisions about where to seek immediate treatment for health issues.

Commercial and government payers, for example, are focused on reducing utilization of hospital-based emergency departments (EDs), claiming EDs are too expensive, make patients wait too long, and allow low-acuity patients to interfere with the care of acutely ill or injured patients. They have increased cost sharing and implemented other reimbursement strategies in an attempt to curb patients' use of the ED. So far,

however, these efforts have failed to reverse the upward trend in utilization.

Through the Emergency Medical Treatment and Active Labor Act (EMTALA) and the "prudent layperson" standard for evaluating whether a patient has an emergency condition, the federal government has mandated that EDs serve as the point of access for anyone who needs medical care. But commercial insurers, and even the Medicaid-serving healthcare intermediaries, have created a quandary by defining many illnesses and injuries as nonemergencies and requiring consumers to pay

About the Author

James J. Augustine, MD, FACEP, is an emergency physician and a member of the American College of Emergency Physicians's board of directors. He is a clinical professor in the Department of Emergency Medicine at Wright State University in Dayton, Ohio, and the chair of the National Clinical Governance Board of US Acute Care Solutions in Canton, Ohio. He also served on The Joint Commission's board of commissioners and chaired its Hospital Professional Technical Advisory Committee. Augustine is the vice president of the Emergency Department Benchmarking Alliance and is a national consultant, author, and speaker on emergency department operations and design.

FUTURESCAN SURVEY RESULTS
Emergency Care

How likely is it that the following will happen by 2023?

Very Likely (%)	Somewhat Likely (%)	Neutral (%)	Somewhat Unlikely (%)	Very Unlikely (%)
23	38	12	22	5

Patient volumes in your hospital's or health system's hospital-based emergency department(s) will increase by more than 10 percent.

Very Likely (%)	Somewhat Likely (%)	Neutral (%)	Somewhat Unlikely (%)	Very Unlikely (%)
20	16	6	22	35

Your hospital or health system will have a freestanding ED located off-site from the hospital campus.

Very Likely (%)	Somewhat Likely (%)	Neutral (%)	Somewhat Unlikely (%)	Very Unlikely (%)
12	41	22	20	6

The number of patients admitted to your hospital or health system from the ED(s) will increase by at least 10 percent.

Very Likely (%)	Somewhat Likely (%)	Neutral (%)	Somewhat Unlikely (%)	Very Unlikely (%)
46	35	10	7	2

Your hospital's or health system's ED(s) will have implemented telemedicine as a means of following up with patients after their visit.

Very Likely (%)	Somewhat Likely (%)	Neutral (%)	Somewhat Unlikely (%)	Very Unlikely (%)
45	16	17	12	10

Your hospital or health system will have employed ED physicians.

Very Likely (%)	Somewhat Likely (%)	Neutral (%)	Somewhat Unlikely (%)	Very Unlikely (%)
24	34	27	11	4

In response to regulatory, market, or insurance pressures, your hospital or health system will have made a price list for emergency services available online, in printed materials, or in the ED(s).

Note: Percentages in each row may not sum exactly to 100% because of rounding.

What Hospital Executives Anticipate by 2023

- Eight in ten leaders (81 percent) think it is at least somewhat likely their emergency department will have implemented telemedicine to follow up with patients after a visit.

- Sixty-one percent say it is somewhat to very likely patient volume will increase by more than 10 percent in their hospital-based ED.

continued on pg. 29

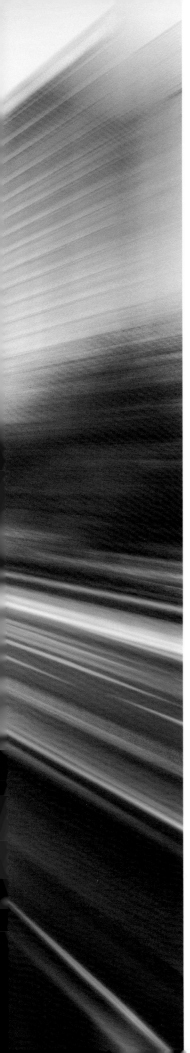

—continued from pg. 27

the entire bill when diagnoses do not meet their reimbursement criteria. Payers characterize this as "surprise billing," which translates into surprise out-of-pocket expenses for patients.

Until recently, there has been little recognition of the patient's need to know what the charges for emergency care will be. That is now changing dramatically in the age of consumerism. The federal government will likely modify EMTALA to allow for the broad and prospective publication of price lists for hospital services, including emergency care. Payers will undoubtedly respond by developing a tiered pricing structure that reduces payments for less acute emergencies and incentivizes patients to seek emergency care from the lowest-priced provider in the region.

Urgent Care Centers

According to the most recent data from the American Academy of Urgent Care Medicine (2017), the number of urgent care centers in the United States has increased from 8,000 in 2008 to more than 9,300 today. Although some urgent care centers are associated with health systems, many are operated by for-profit chains and physician groups.

In the coming years, health systems across the country, along with other entities, will continue to build urgent care centers in locations where convenient, lower-cost services will fulfill a regional need. In some cases, this will occur because a hospital (or its ED) will have reached its limit for patient volume or have insufficient access to primary care than is necessary to serve community needs.

Urgent care centers can also serve as the site of follow-up care for patients who are seen in hospital EDs, have restricted access to primary care, or require ongoing care for a chronic medical condition.

Walk-In Clinics

The market has also seen an explosion of walk-in clinics. In 2018, the number of such clinics is projected to surpass 2,800 nationwide, according to research by Accenture (2015).

This number reflects a 47 percent increase over 2014, when 1,914 walk-in clinics existed.

In addition to large clinic operators such as CVS, Walgreens, and Walmart, a growing number of health systems are getting into the act by partnering with retailers to offer consumers walk-in convenience for basic health services, which often are paid out of pocket.

Freestanding Emergency Departments

Over the past decade, freestanding emergency departments (FSEDs) have emerged as a new option to meet the need for convenient care. They are designed to fill geographic and service gaps, offer a lower-volume (and lower-cost) approach to emergency care, generate outpatient revenue, and drive inpatient volumes. In addition to those operated by local and regional health systems, some FSEDs are operated by for-profit entities.

According to Harvard University researchers, there are currently more than 500 FSEDs in the United States (Morrison 2016). Regulations for these facilities vary by state, but only one state, California, specifically precludes them. Arizona, Colorado, Minnesota, Ohio, and Texas have the most FSEDs per capita. If these early adopters are emulated by other states where regulators allow them, there could be as many as 2,000 in the near future (Morrison 2016).

Some providers and health policy experts are concerned that FSED chains will attract the most desirable patients and payers, leaving community hospitals with the unsustainable burden of providing more charity care in their EDs.

Conversely, FSEDs operated by health systems can treat low-acuity patients and transfer those with more severe illnesses and injuries to their hospital-based EDs, thus providing a viable business model for the systems. At this point, relatively few leaders participating in the *Futurescan* national survey expect to employ this strategy in the near future. Only 20 percent say their organization will have an FSED located off-site from the hospital campus by 2023.

continued from pg. 28

- Nearly half (45 percent) of respondents believe it is very likely their hospital or health system will employ ED physicians. Another 16 percent think it is somewhat likely.

- Fifty-eight percent say it is at least somewhat likely they will have a publicly available price list for emergency services.

Microhospitals

Also new to the field are microhospitals with an ED—small-scale, inpatient facilities that provide around-the-clock care to low-acuity patients and must conform to the same federal and state licensing requirements and regulations as conventional hospitals. Typically, microhospitals range in size from 15,000 to 50,000 square feet and have between eight and ten inpatient beds for observation and short-term stays. The

facilities also frequently house ancillary services and primary care physician offices.

No two microhospitals are exactly the same in their design or service mix, but one trend is clear: A growing number of health systems are developing them as entry points into markets where demand does not support larger, more comprehensive hospitals. Currently, microhospitals can be found in 19 states (Mirza 2017).

Telemedicine

Telemedicine continues to gain traction, driven by the rise in consumerism and the need to deliver care in remote areas. In emergency medicine, hospitals and health systems are increasingly using the technology to provide the following:

- An alternative to going to the ED and a convenient way for patients to access a doctor quickly via smartphones and software platforms that make it easier to connect patients with providers
- An efficient way to follow up with patients after an emergency visit

- A means to offer emergency care in medically underserved areas that lack nearby access to a hospital
- An option for ED physicians to consult with off-site radiologists or specialists about stroke, trauma, and critical care cases, as well as other complex patient conditions

Payers are also playing a key role in advancing the technology, exploring telemedicine as an economical way to deliver low-acuity, episodic care. Some insurance companies have even begun steering patients away from urgent care and other facilities to telemedicine options.

Hospital Emergency Departments

Although many other options for immediate and emergency care are now available to consumers, they have not reduced the number of patient visits to hospitals. In fact, more people are visiting EDs than ever before.

Since 1992, volumes have steadily grown about 2.5 percent annually and are expected to continue to increase for the foreseeable future (Gindi, Black, and Cohen 2016). Why do the numbers continue to rise despite the heightened competition?

Part of the answer lies in the nation's demographics. Members of the baby boom generation are beginning to reach the age when they require more medical services, including the ED.

Other factors are identified in the results of the Centers for Disease Control and Prevention's annual National Hospital Ambulatory Medical Care

Survey on the reasons patients seek emergency care (CDC 2017):

- Many patients with commercial insurance simply prefer to use a hospital ED after hours when their doctor's office is closed.
- Medicaid patients often choose the ED because they are concerned the medical issue they have is serious.
- The uninsured tend to choose the ED because they lack access to other providers.

Executives responding to the *Futurescan* survey are less certain about the growth projections, with only 23 percent saying it is very likely patient volumes in their hospital-based emergency department will increase by more than 10 percent in the next five years.

Implications for the Future

As hospital and health system leaders focus on positioning their organizations for success in the new era of emergency medicine, they should consider the following action steps:

- Understand the impact of consumerism and retailization on the field. Realize that patients' expectations are influenced by their experiences with other industries, including anytime/anywhere availability and more personalized, self-directed services.
- Be aware that competition is happening on many fronts, and proactively explore new models for enhancing the quality, cost, and timeliness of emergency care (e.g., FSEDs, microhospitals, the expansion of urgent care centers). Determine whether the best strategy for your organization is to compete, to collaborate, or to innovate if it is to maintain a strong market position and seize new opportunities.
- Develop pricing and transparency policies that enhance the perceived value of emergency services, and clarify pricing and billing practices.
- Recognize and adapt to the shifting trends and pressures from payers and government regulators.

> Consumers are increasingly demanding emergency care when and how they want it. Ever more sensitive to cost and value, patients are playing a more proactive role in choosing how their healthcare dollar is spent.

- Prepare for the projected continued increase in hospital ED volumes.
- Dedicate the resources needed for the effective delivery of emergency care in the changing environment.
- Adjust to the reality that a range of diagnostic and treatment services traditionally delivered only in the ED are now available in other (e.g., ambulatory, community, virtual) settings.

In addition to preparing for these trends, leaders must remain focused on their mission moving forward. Hospitals will continue to serve as the front line and safety net for our healthcare system and the millions of Americans, both insured and uninsured, who rely on them daily for emergency care.

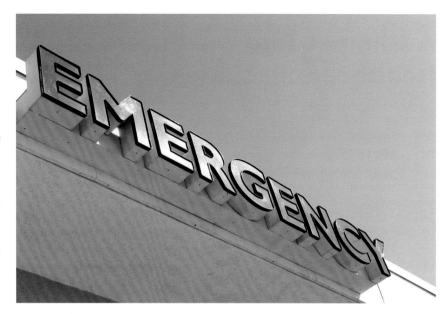

References

Accenture. 2015. "Number of US Retail Clinics Will Surpass 2,800 by 2017, Accenture Forecasts." Published November 12. https://newsroom.accenture.com/news/number-of-us-retail-health-clinics-will-surpass-2800-by-2017-accenture-forecasts.htm.

American Academy of Urgent Care Medicine. 2017. "Future of Urgent Care." Accessed November 10. http://aaucm.org/about/future/.

Centers for Disease Control and Prevention (CDC). 2017. "National Hospital Ambulatory Medical Care Survey: 2014 Emergency Department Summary Tables." Published September. https://www.cdc.gov/nchs/data/nhamcs/web_tables/2014_ed_web_tables.pdf.

Gindi, R.M., L.I. Black, and R.A. Cohen. 2016. "Reasons for Emergency Room Use Among US Adults Aged 18–64: National Health Interview Survey, 2013 and 2014." National Health Statistics Report 90. Published February 18. https://www.cdc.gov/nchs/data/nhsr/nhsr090.pdf.

Mirza, A. 2017. "Micro-hospitals Provide Health Care Closer to Home." *U.S. News & World Report*. Published April 24. www.usnews.com/news/healthcare-of-tomorrow/articles/2017-04-24/micro-hospitals-offer-an-alternative-health-care-model-for-local-communities.

Morrison, I. 2016. "The Future of Emergency Care." *Hospitals & Health Networks*. Published November 7. www.hhnmag.com/articles/7795-the-future-of-emergency-care.

A Glimpse into the Future of Healthcare Facilities

by Don King

The transformation of healthcare, the need for resiliency, and escalating safety and security concerns are requiring leaders to reengineer and reimagine medical facilities in ways that will profoundly affect where care and other services are delivered in the future.

The Shift Away from the Traditional Model

Although the hospital remains the epicenter of many health systems, advances in medicine, a growing emphasis on cost reduction, and the continued trend toward population health are increasingly driving organizations to move away from the hospital-centric model via two strategies:

1. **Acquiring or renting off-site locations.** In this year's *Futurescan* survey, 34 percent of healthcare leaders said it is very likely their hospital or health system will acquire off-site, nonhealthcare facilities for outpatient services. Another 37 percent said it is somewhat likely. Conveniently, just as healthcare organizations are seeking remote locations that are large enough to house clinics, surgical centers, and rehabilitation facilities, many major retailers are discovering that their bricks-and-mortar stores are simply untenable given the growth in online consumer shopping (Gesenhues 2017; Kestenbaum 2017). As a result, vast amounts of affordable commercial space are available to healthcare providers.

These properties tend to be in the heart of communities and thus within short driving or walking distance of residential developments and businesses. They were designed for convenience, with ample parking and easy access to public transportation. Furthermore, their high ceilings make them perfect for large medical equipment. In short, they are ideal for dispersed healthcare facilities.

2. **Repurposing hospitals.** Declining inpatient volumes and the migration of medical services away from a main campus sometimes result in hospital relocations or closures (*Becker's Hospital Review* 2017). To address the problem, leaders are increasingly repurposing former hospital space. The Detroit Medical Center, for example, has converted the former Hutzel Women's Hospital into administrative offices and an updated Ronald McDonald House (Galbraith 2015). Other hospitals have used available space on often-sprawling former hospital campuses to develop freestanding cancer care centers, medical fitness complexes, and physician office buildings.

In addition to healthcare organizations, third-party developers often take on adaptive-reuse projects. A developer in New Jersey, for instance, has purchased abandoned hospitals in Paterson, Jersey City,

About the Author

Don King is the president of Donald King Consulting, which provides healthcare organizations with strategic programs for plant operations, maintenance, and energy. For more than 40 years, he has worked with organizations in the private sector, academic medical centers, and government health systems to improve the safety, effectiveness, and efficiency of their facilities. He previously served as director of facilities for the University of Michigan Medical Center and vice president of facilities operations for Kaiser Permanente. King graduated with honors from Cleary University and holds certifications as a healthcare facility manager and a business energy professional. He currently chairs the National Fire Protection Association's committee on medical equipment and serves as lead for the Healthcare Executive Leadership Council of the American Society for Healthcare Engineering, a professional membership group of the American Hospital Association.

FUTURESCAN SURVEY RESULTS
Facilities

How likely is it that the following will happen by 2023?

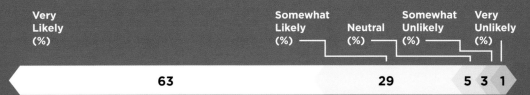

Very Likely (%)	Somewhat Likely (%)	Neutral (%)	Somewhat Unlikely (%)	Very Unlikely (%)
63	29	5	3	1

Your hospital or health system will have made capital investments to redesign or equip existing facilities in ways that improve patient and staff safety.

| 63 | 28 | 6 | 2 | 1 |

Your hospital or health system will have installed surveillance and alarm systems in high-risk areas, such as pharmacies, parking lots, or cash-handling locations.

| 51 | 32 | 11 | 5 | 1 |

Your hospital or health system will have invested in networked security systems that support high-definition surveillance cameras.

| 36 | 37 | 17 | 8 | 2 |

Your hospital or health system will have made capital investments in the design or redesign of facilities to enhance resiliency (the capacity to adapt to changing conditions and to maintain or regain functionality in the face of stress or disaster) and prevent disruptions to patient care.

| 34 | 37 | 14 | 10 | 5 |

Your hospital or health system will have acquired and repurposed off-site non-healthcare facilities (e.g., retail or commercial office space) for outpatient services.

Note: Percentages in each row may not sum exactly to 100% because of rounding.

What Hospital Executives Anticipate by 2023

- Nearly two-thirds (63 percent) believe it is very likely their hospital or health system will have installed surveillance and alarm systems in high-risk areas. Another 28 percent say it is somewhat likely.

- Sixty-three percent of respondents say it is very likely their organization will have made capital investments to improve patient and staff safety.

- Eighty-three percent think it is at least somewhat likely they will have purchased a high-definition networked surveillance system.

- Seven in ten respondents (71 percent) say it is somewhat to very likely their organization will have acquired and repurposed off-site nonhealthcare facilities to provide outpatient services.

—continued from pg. 32

Hammonton, and Trenton and converted them into medical malls that offer a myriad of services (Kaysen 2014).

Rule that took effect in 2017 requires healthcare providers to have a plan in place to deal with equipment and power failures, loss of part or all of their facilities, and interruptions in

American women it has escalated from 15 percent in 1980 to 35 percent in 2015 (GBD Obesity Collaborators 2017). This increases the potential risk of injuries among hospital staff who care for heavier patients. In 2015, nongovernment hospitals reported six nonfatal occupational injuries or illnesses per 100 employees, compared with three for all nongovernment workplaces (US Bureau of Labor Statistics 2016).

> Advances in medicine, a growing emphasis on cost reduction, and the continued trend toward population health are increasingly driving organizations to move away from the hospital-centric model.

The convergence of these trends is reflected in the five-year capital plan of the University of New Mexico Health Sciences, which includes building a replacement hospital, repurposing the old hospital for teaching and faculty spaces, and repurposing several on-campus buildings, as well as the construction of numerous community-based clinics (University of New Mexico 2017).

Improving Resiliency

The *Futurescan* survey also showed that many hospitals are investing in the design or redesign of facilities to improve their resiliency. Thirty-six percent of respondents indicated they are very likely to make such investments within the next five years, and 37 percent said they are somewhat likely to do so.

The greater focus on resiliency is the result of two factors:

1. **An increase in natural disasters.** The frequency and severity of hurricanes, tornadoes, storms, floods, and earthquakes are on the rise, causing billions of dollars in damage to medical facilities across the nation. Hospitals must not only withstand such disasters but also be fully capable of dealing with a possible surge in patient volume.
2. **New government regulations.** The Centers for Medicare & Medicaid Services Emergency Preparedness

communications, such as those from cyber attacks (CMS 2017).

Other government regulations have been in place for years. Perhaps the best known is the California seismic safety requirement mandating that, by 2030, all hospitals in the state be able to operate at full capacity after a major earthquake (California Hospital Association 2011).

Ensuring Safety and Security

The *Futurescan* survey asked three questions related to safety and security, and the majority of respondents indicated they would be taking action to improve both. Specifically, 63 percent said it is very likely their hospital or health system will make capital investments to redesign or equip existing facilities in ways that improve patient and staff safety; 63 percent said it is very likely they will install surveillance and alarm systems in high-risk areas, such as pharmacies, parking lots, or cash-handling locations; and 51 percent said it is very likely they will invest in networked security systems that support high-definition surveillance cameras.

The heightened attention to investments in safety and security is being driven by the following trends:

- **An increase in staff injuries.** The prevalence of obesity among American men has risen from 11 percent in 1980 to 31 percent in 2015, and among

- **The price of drugs.** While narcotics such as oxycodone have attracted thieves for years, some recently developed nonnarcotic medications commonly stored in hospital pharmacies may also become prime targets. For example, Harvoni, approved by the Food and Drug Administration to fight hepatitis C, costs nearly $95,000 for a 12-week regimen, and Ilaris, used to treat patients with rare inflammatory disorders and heart attacks, costs $16,000 per dose. Both drugs are considered easy to resell on the street.
- **The threat of violence.** As the world grows more dangerous, the incidence of violence in healthcare settings is on the rise—putting patients, visitors, physicians, and staff at risk (OSHA 2015). According to The Joint Commission, violent crimes in hospitals have risen from two such events per 100 beds in 2012 to almost three in 2015 (Stempniak 2017). In addition, the Federal Bureau of Investigation identified at least seven "active shooter" incidents in US medical facilities between 2001 and 2016 (FBI 2016).

Implications for Healthcare Organizations

The issues and trends highlighted here have major implications for hospitals and health systems seeking to expand or update their facilities.

Off-site facilities. An off-site facilities strategy requires serious long-term planning and consideration of all the potential ramifications. Buying existing buildings that were previously used by retailers will not necessarily be less expensive than developing a new healthcare facility, unless the real estate market in that area is significantly depressed. A recent study of Seattle Children's South Clinic indicated that renovating vacant retail space into an outpatient facility is only 2 percent cheaper than the cost of new construction (Hansen 2017; Miller, Saga, and Nichols 2016). Whatever the purchase price, the acquired buildings will probably require extensive remodeling to bring them up to healthcare standards.

An example is the Midway Clinic, which is part of HealthEast, a four-hospital organization in Minnesota. Midway Clinic originally opened in 1983 in Saint Paul but moved in 2012 from a leased space into a former Borders bookstore only a few blocks away. The space was totally reconfigured to enable the clinic to add more medical specialties and services. The former bookstore's spacious parking lot and central location were key draws. "We chose the new site because of its convenience for patients," said Len Kaiser, director of business development for HealthEast clinics. "It has plenty of free parking, is easily accessible from the freeway, and there are other amenities nearby" (HealthEast Care System 2012).

Off-site buildings require dispersed administration and facilities management. The additional work and duplication of services and equipment necessary to maintain offices away from the main campus should not be underestimated. Often it means dealing with a third-party landlord and working with the owner to address the special needs of a healthcare facility, including backup power, fire safety, and other issues. A careful study of the neighborhood is also crucial to ensure nearby businesses are compatible with the mission of a hospital or health system.

Hospital repurposing. As some hospitals relocate or close, vacated buildings and open campus land become opportunities for repurposing to house clinical services that may be better suited to the sites. The populations served should be carefully analyzed so that their daily routines can be determined and their access

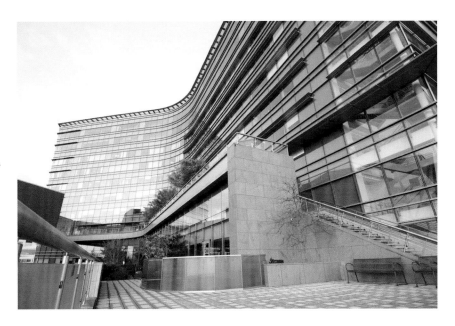

to healthcare optimized. Acknowledging this trend, the state of Maryland passed Senate Bill 707 exempting hospitals from the certificate-of-need process when converting a licensed general hospital into a freestanding medical facility (General Assembly of Maryland 2017).

Leaders should also consider whether these spaces can be effectively used for nonclinical functions or transformed into retail-based healthcare complexes by third-party developers. Ultimately, deciding the best use for vacant medical campuses should be part of a hospital's or health system's strategic and facilities planning process led by the executive team and board of directors in conjunction with the neighboring community and local municipal officials.

Resiliency requirements. The need to protect against natural catastrophes will tax many healthcare organizations' budgets. For example, the California Hospital Association (2011) estimated that it will cost hospitals $110 billion to meet the state's earthquake resiliency requirements. Hospitals in areas at risk for hurricanes, storm flooding, and wildfires will also need to take steps to increase the resiliency of their facilities to prepare for these disasters. These include evaluating the design of critical structures, moving essential services and equipment to higher ground, having adequate backup emergency generators, and installing

storm-resistant roofs and windows. Healthcare organizations' dependence on technology increases the importance of resiliency in information technology systems, as well as in the power and water utilities that support them.

Caregiver safety. In addition to providing quality care to patients, hospitals and health systems must protect the health and safety of caregivers. For example, as obesity rates rise, organizations will need to purchase lift devices and special equipment to help nurses and other staff safely move larger patients without putting themselves at risk of injury (NIDDKD 2017). Doorways and hallways in healthcare facilities may need to be widened to accommodate bigger wheelchairs.

Pharmaceutical security. Hospitals have long been required to keep narcotics safely stored. In the future, both hospital-based and off-site outpatient pharmacies may need to extend the same precautions to other drugs that are in demand on the street by increasing their investment in theft prevention equipment, such as security cameras and alarms, along with the advanced data-handling capabilities that such equipment requires. Hospitals with outdated information technology networks will need major upgrades to accommodate the volume of data from this equipment, not to mention data from electronic health records, networked medical devices, and other connected sources.

Violence prevention. To protect against the increased risk of violence, hospital leaders must establish emergency communication systems and procedures, create control centers and safe rooms, install automatic locking devices on doors and elevators, and train hospital security officers and staff at all levels of the organization on how to deal with violent incidents (Kendig and Mykoo 2012). Some hospitals are choosing to deploy real-time location systems that not only track employees' movements but also can be used to trigger alarms and provide precise location information in emergency situations.

Conclusion

Clearly, the new era of healthcare requires greater forethought and planning for hospital and health system facilities. Leaders must assemble a team that is highly skilled in building construction, design, operations, and maintenance—as well as outside experts in architecture, engineering, and real estate—to develop effective strategies to address the trends outlined here. Those who do so will ensure their organizations are well positioned to face future facilities challenges and opportunities.

References

Becker's Hospital Review. 2017. "6 Thoughts on the Movement from Inpatient to Outpatient Care." Published February 8. www.beckershospitalreview.com/hospital-management-administration/6-thoughts-on-the-movement-from-inpatient-to-outpatient-care.html.

California Hospital Association. 2011. "Earthquake-Compliant Hospital Buildings vs. Access to Care: California's Careful Balancing Act." Published March. www.calhospital.org/issue-paper/earthquake-compliant-hospital-buildings-vs-access-care-californias-careful-balancing-act.

Centers for Medicare & Medicaid Services (CMS). 2017. "Emergency Preparedness Rule." Published October 4. www.cms.gov/Medicare/Provider-Enrollment-and-Certification/SurveyCertEmergPrep/Emergency-PrepRule.html.

Federal Bureau of Investigation (FBI). 2016. "Active Shooter Incidents in the United States from 2000–2016." Published September 8. www.fbi.gov/file-repository/activeshooter_incidents_2001-2016.pdf.

Galbraith, M.J. 2015. "Repurposing Historic Buildings on Detroit's Medical Campuses." Model D Media. Published July 14. www.modeldmedia.com/features/historic-preservation-hospitals-071415.aspx.

GBD Obesity Collaborators. 2017. Supplementary appendix to "Health Effects of Overweight and Obesity in 195 Countries over 25 Years." *New England Journal of Medicine* 377 (1): 13–27. Accessed July 20. www.nejm.org/doi/suppl/10.1056/NEJMoa1614362/suppl_file/nejmoa1614362_appendix.pdf.

General Assembly of Maryland. 2017. "Freestanding Medical Facilities—Certificate of Need, Rates, and Definition." Published October 24. http://mgaleg.maryland.gov/webmga/frmMain.aspx?id=sb0707&stab=01&pid=billpage&tab=subject3&ys=2016rs.

Gesenhues, A. 2017. "Report: E-commerce Accounted for 11.7% of Total Retail Sales in 2016, Up 15.6% over 2015." *Marketing Land*. Published February 20. http://marketingland.com/report-e-commerce-accounted-11-7-total-retail-sales-2016-15-6-2015-207088.

Hansen, M. 2017. "From Big Box to Clinic: Seattle Children's South Clinic." Presentation at the 2017 American Society for Healthcare Engineering PDC Summit, Orlando, FL, March 13.

HealthEast Care System. 2012. "New HealthEast Midway Clinic Is Open." *Compass*. Published April. www.myhealthnewsletter.com/healtheast/April12/article2.html.

Kaysen, R. 2014. "Repurposing Closed Hospitals as For-Profit Medical Malls." *New York Times*. Published March 4. www.nytimes.com/2014/03/05/realestate/commercial/repurposing-closed-hospitals-as-for-profit-medical-malls.html.

Kendig, J., and Y. Mykoo. 2012. "Active Shooters in the Hospital Environment." Presentation to the Florida Department of Health. Accessed July 20, 2017. www.floridahealth.gov/programs-and-services/emergency-preparedness-and-response/_documents/active-shooter.pdf.

Kestenbaum, R. 2017. "Why So Many Stores Are Closing Now." *Forbes*. Published April 7. www.forbes.com/sites/richardkestenbaum/2017/04/07/why-so-many-stores-are-closing-now/.

Miller, S., T. Saga, and V. Nichols. 2016. "From Big Box Retail to Community Clinic: How Adaptive Reuse Opened the Door for Seattle Children's Newest Clinic." *Inside ASHE*. Published March. www.nxtbook.com/naylor/ ENVQ/ENVQ0116/index.php?startid=38#/40.

National Institute of Diabetes and Digestive and Kidney Diseases (NIDDKD). 2017. "Overweight and Obesity Statistics." Published August. www.niddk.nih.gov/health-information/health-statistics/overweight-obesity.

Occupational Safety and Health Administration (OSHA). 2015. "Workplace Violence in Healthcare: Understanding the Challenge." Accessed July 20, 2017. www.osha.gov/Publications/OSHA3826.pdf.

Stempniak, M. 2017. "Violence in the Hospital: Preventing Assaults Using a Clinical Approach." *Hospitals & Health Networks*. Published June 9. www.hhnmag.com/articles/8306-violence-in-the-hospital-preventing-assaults-using-a-clinical-approach.

University of New Mexico. 2017. "Five-Year Capital Plan: Health Sciences Center." Published August 8. http://pdc.unm.edu/strategic-leadership/capital-planning/5-year-capital-list.pdf.

US Bureau of Labor Statistics. 2016. "Table 1. Incidence Rates of Nonfatal Occupational Injuries and Illnesses by Case Type and Ownership, Selected Industries, 2015." Published October 27. www.bls.gov/news.release/osh.t01.htm.

Purchaser Pressure: The Emerging Role of Employers in Driving Value in Healthcare

by David Lansky, PhD

As medical costs consume an ever-increasing share of businesses' profits, self-funded employers and public purchasers of health insurance are becoming more aggressive than ever before in direct contracting with providers.

Their heightened interest in this strategy is the result of growing dissatisfaction with insurers' lack of progress in improving the value of healthcare. Employers have found that working directly with physicians and hospitals creates opportunities to

- improve the quality of patient care and outcomes,
- enhance the patient experience,
- increase price transparency,
- steer employees to narrow provider networks, and
- manage costs more predictably.

For example, the Cleveland Clinic, Johns Hopkins Medicine, and the Employers Centers of Excellence Network offer travel surgery programs that allow employees from large companies such as Walmart to receive high-quality, appropriate care with no out-of-pocket costs (Johns Hopkins Medicine 2015; Slotkin et al. 2017; Zeltner 2012). And a number of large employers, including Boeing and Intel, have had success in contracting directly with provider organizations to manage the health of an enrolled population, leading to rapid improvements in the providers' quality performance and predictable multiyear costs (DeVore and Cates 2015; Evans 2015; Mecklenburg 2016).

How Much Will Employers Push the Market?

Despite the initial successes, significant barriers impede more widespread adoption of direct contracting:

- Employers value the one-stop shopping that working with a comprehensive health plan provides.
- Employers prefer a "hands-off" relationship when it comes to decisions about their employees' provider network and access.
- Businesses do not have the bandwidth to build a complete network and negotiate numerous contracts.
- Most companies do not have the competence or confidence to evaluate and oversee direct provider relationships.
- Employers believe few healthcare organizations are capable of assuming risk and orchestrating complex care arrangements.

About the Author
David Lansky, PhD, is president and CEO of the Pacific Business Group on Health, where he directs efforts to improve the affordability and availability of high-quality healthcare. Since 2008, he has led the coalition of 60 large employers and healthcare purchasers that represent more than 10 million Americans and include Wells Fargo, Intel, Safeway, Walmart, Boeing, CalPERS, and the Washington State Health Care Authority. A nationally recognized expert on accountability, quality measurement, and health information technology, Lansky has served as a board member or adviser to numerous healthcare programs, including the National Quality Forum, Joint Commission, and Leapfrog Group. He is the current chair of the Health Care Transformation Task Force industry consortium, and he also serves on the guiding committee of the US Department of Health & Human Services Health Care Payment Learning & Action Network, the health advisers panel of the Congressional Budget Office, and the board of the Alliance for Health Policy.

FUTURESCAN SURVEY RESULTS
Role of Employers

How likely is it that the following will happen by 2023?

Very Likely (%)	Somewhat Likely (%)	Neutral (%)	Somewhat Unlikely (%)	Very Unlikely (%)
27	33	18	11	12

At least 10 percent of your hospital's or health system's total revenue from patient care will come from direct contracts with self-funded employers.

Very Likely (%)	Somewhat Likely (%)	Neutral (%)	Somewhat Unlikely (%)	Very Unlikely (%)
15	30	31	18	6

At least 20 percent of your hospital's or health system's total revenue from total joint replacement surgery will come from bundled payments.

Very Likely (%)	Somewhat Likely (%)	Neutral (%)	Somewhat Unlikely (%)	Very Unlikely (%)
56	29	8	4	4

Your hospital or health system will have routinely collected patient-reported outcome measures for services such as total joint replacement, cardiac surgery, cancer treatment, or mental health care to assess patients' health status.

Very Likely (%)	Somewhat Likely (%)	Neutral (%)	Somewhat Unlikely (%)	Very Unlikely (%)
1	8	16	22	54

Your hospital or health system will have operated a freestanding birthing center that accounts for at least 20 percent of your low-risk births.

Very Likely (%)	Somewhat Likely (%)	Neutral (%)	Somewhat Unlikely (%)	Very Unlikely (%)
40	36	16	7	2

Your hospital or health system will participate in a regional health information exchange that shares emergency department and admissions data with health plans and other risk-bearing provider organizations.

Very Likely (%)	Somewhat Likely (%)	Neutral (%)	Somewhat Unlikely (%)	Very Unlikely (%)
8	21	23	29	20

At least 10 percent of your hospital's or health system's current inpatient facility space will be converted to provide community wellness and well-being services.

Note: Percentages in each row may not sum exactly to 100% because of rounding.

What Hospital Executives Anticipate by 2023

- Six in ten leaders (60 percent) believe it is at least somewhat likely that a minimum of 10 percent of their total patient care revenue will come from contracts with self-funded employers.

continued on pg. 40

—continued from pg. 38

Nonetheless, I believe the trend toward direct contracting between employers and providers will grow slowly but persistently. In the latest *Futurescan* survey, 60 percent of participating hospital and health system leaders indicated it is somewhat to very likely that at least a tenth of their total revenue will come from these kinds of contracts by 2023.

I also anticipate that there will continue to be strong interest in direct arrangements with accountable care organizations (ACOs), as well as increased use of episode-based payments and direct contracts for spine, maternity, cancer, and

features, reflecting the experiences and values that employers bring to the market.

Accountability for quality. Leading businesses will increasingly select providers on the basis of quality, outcome, cost, and utilization data as they strive to offer their employees the best possible care while controlling overall medical expenses. Employer-sponsored ACOs and bundled-payment arrangements generally have higher quality standards than do those sponsored by commercial health plans. Employers also frequently evaluate the performance of individual

To support this focus on quality, most employers expect the providers they partner with to commit to adopting fully capable electronic health records and clinical information systems and to join appropriate clinical registries. In fact, three-quarters of *Futurescan* survey respondents said they are at least somewhat likely to be involved in a data exchange with health plans and other caregivers in the next five years, particularly to track admissions and emergency department visits across their community.

New financial arrangements. Employers' direct contracts with providers are built on new reimbursement models and new approaches to consumer incentives. Companies are looking for predictable, multiyear, total-cost-of-care contracts that are based on either a global budget for a population or a prospectively determined price for an episode of care.

> Leading businesses will increasingly select providers on the basis of quality, outcome, cost, and utilization data as they strive to offer their employees the best possible care while controlling overall medical expenses.

orthopedic care. This, too, is supported by the survey results: A significant number of executives predict that, within the next five years, bundled payments will account for more than 20 percent of their total joint replacement surgery income.

What to Expect in the Future

Moving forward, new employer-driven contracting and payment arrangements are likely to have several common

providers to be included in a preferred network.

For example, the Employers Centers of Excellence Network travel surgery program only qualifies orthopedic surgeons from distinguished hospitals that have a strong track record in delivering safe, effective care and an exceptional patient experience. Notably, 85 percent of healthcare executives participating in the *Futurescan* survey said they are somewhat to very likely to routinely collect such measures by 2023.

Many health plans have trouble administering these models and prefer to offer products that build on the existing fee-for-service claims payment systems they operate at scale. This is one area where physicians, hospitals, and other healthcare organizations can establish a more responsive and accountable relationship with the employer customer. Businesses will expect providers to assume financial risk in meeting negotiated budget targets for total spending for an enrolled or attributed population; providers will both have an opportunity to capture savings when they outperform the target and risk losses if they fail to meet it.

For episodes of care, employers also prefer contracts with prospectively

continued from pg. 39

- Fifty-six percent think it is very likely their hospital or health system will routinely collect patient-reported outcome measures, and another 29 percent consider it somewhat likely.

- Three-quarters (76 percent) say it is at least somewhat likely their organization will participate in a regional health information exchange to share emergency department and admissions data with health plans and other risk-bearing providers.

- Almost half (45 percent) of respondents believe it is somewhat to very likely that at least 20 percent of revenue from total joint replacement surgeries will come from bundled payments.

negotiated prices that reflect the total cost of care across all services and providers. Today, most purchasers accept that they must negotiate shared-savings approaches as a first step toward shifting providers into taking on risk and entering into direct contracts; however, they ultimately expect that a competitive market will produce efficiencies that return all savings to the patient and employer—the ultimate payers.

These shared-savings models will not be based solely on efficiencies; employers feel strongly about their moral and fiduciary responsibility to their workers and their workers' families and will not distribute financial gains until the contracted providers have passed mutually agreed-upon quality thresholds. Often these standards will reflect specific concerns of employers or their communities.

Community collaboration. Businesses know that their employees' health is only partly dependent on medical care. Increasingly, they are looking for providers who can help promote the well-being of the whole person, including understanding and addressing the social determinants of health, engaging in community partnerships, and using the workplace as a venue for health education and support.

They want their provider partners to deliver effective workplace-based health programs, such as on-site clinics, wellness and disease management offerings, and telehealth, as well as social welfare, mental health, and other community services.

Many businesses express frustration at the slow rate of progress in addressing important health issues for their employees—for example, managing diabetes, diagnosing and treating lower back pain, increasing appropriate birthing options, eliminating unnecessary cesarean sections, and helping people overcome depression.

To combat the problem, payers and purchasers in some communities have identified health priorities and incorporated performance requirements in their contracts to focus providers on

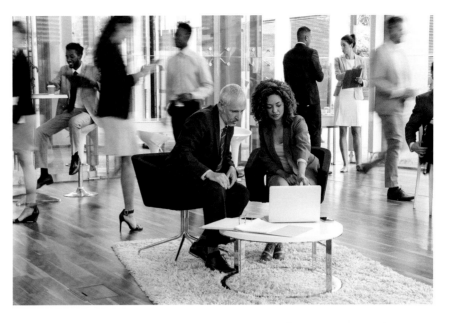

improving care in these areas. They have done so by specifying medical best practices and implementing communitywide measurement and benchmarking.

Specific examples include the following:

- The Covered California health insurance exchange has established health improvement targets in its contracts with providers (Heartland Institute 2016).
- The state of Washington's public employee program ACO contracts take advantage of the standards developed by a regional multistakeholder group (Bree Collaborative 2017).
- Intel's ACO contract with providers emphasizes improved diabetes care (DeVore and Cates 2015).

Favorable conditions for employer direct contracting. Will these approaches come into play in your area? In reality, many of these initiatives will happen slowly and inconsistently across the country. They are more likely to become viable in markets with the following enabling characteristics:

- *A small number of purchasers sponsor a significant proportion of the commercial insurance covered lives in a region.* In such markets, purchasers are often large companies or state agencies. In Seattle, Boeing covers more than

100,000 lives in a region with a population of about 4 million. Intel achieved similar buying influence in Albuquerque with only 4,000 lives in a population-based contract.
- *There is alignment and collaboration between big local employers and public purchasers.* The Arkansas Medicaid program has worked closely with Walmart on the design of its bundled-payment and medical home programs.
- *Providers are ready to take on risk and be accountable for delivering high-quality care.* Intel was able to work with the Presbyterian Health System in Albuquerque and Qualcomm could negotiate a partnership with Scripps Health in San Diego because the organizations had previously worked hard to build integrated, coordinated, and accountable systems of care to satisfy other market requirements, such as Medicare Advantage contracting.

Implications for Healthcare Leaders
As businesses assume a larger role in shaping the way healthcare is purchased and delivered in the United States, hospitals and health systems must be prepared for the new market dynamics. Following are steps leaders can take to position their organizations for future success.

Determine your readiness. Begin the internal conversation about where you are best able to assume risk or offer bundled pricing. Compile performance data on your priority service lines or population to gauge your readiness to participate in the new pricing and quality models. And understand how you compare to regional or out-of-market competitors.

Talk to regional employers. Engage with employers and business associations in your market to find out what they are looking for from physicians, hospitals, and health systems; how they evaluate providers; and what consumer incentives they will offer employees to enroll in new networks. Identify the largest local companies and the major national employers with a big footprint in your area to see if they are seeking partners in value-based contracting. Keep in mind that more than 50 regional business coalitions understand these models and are available to help broker relationships between interested employers and capable providers (National Alliance of Healthcare Purchaser Coalitions 2017).

Reap the benefits of value-based care. Employers rely on economist Michael Porter's formula for healthcare in developing direct contracts with providers: *Value = patient health outcomes ÷ the total cost of care* (Porter and Lee 2013). The increased focus on reporting outcomes, along with the new population- and episode-based payment models that require measuring aggregate medical expenses over time, will provide

companies with the tools needed to implement the formula. Take advantage of the benefits that a health insurance market driven by value and competition offers, including less micromonitoring of care processes, more opportunity for innovation, and better outcomes at lower costs with novel uses of your workforce, technology, or sites of care.

A good example is bundled payment for maternity care. Many companies do not want to pay providers more for performing cesarean sections than vaginal births or for delivering babies in the hospital instead of in birthing centers; they want providers to make greater use of midwives, doulas, and other less invasive options (de Brantes and Love 2016; Health Care Payment Learning & Action Network 2016). In the *Futurescan* survey, only 9 percent of healthcare executives said they are somewhat to very likely to operate a freestanding birthing center that accounts for at least 20 percent of their low-risk births in the next five years. But providers would be wise to listen to their employer customers and look more closely at ways to reduce costs while achieving the same or better outcomes (Stapleton, Osborne, and Illuzzi 2013; Woo et al. 2017).

Engage in regional efforts. Most communities today have created organizations to help providers collaborate on the necessary infrastructure for accountable care without building everything themselves. Health information exchanges, data warehouses and all-payer claims systems, quality improvement resources, and common measurement

and benchmarking are all candidates for collective investment rather than competition. A number of multipayer initiatives are also emerging that intend to standardize payment methods so that all providers have consistent incentives. Your region may be part of a Centers for Medicare & Medicaid Services State Innovation Models grant, mandatory joint replacement bundle initiative, or Comprehensive Primary Care Plus demonstration that could provide a focus for direct contracting. You can accelerate the shift to value-based payment and take advantage of the chance to work directly with purchasers by helping to build a more efficient community structure for provider competition.

Conclusion

In these challenging times, employers are driving vital changes in healthcare by

- promoting new, disruptive models of care and reimbursement;
- fostering innovations that improve quality and lower costs;
- facilitating vital community partnerships; and
- demanding increased accountability from all stakeholders involved.

Ultimately, these will be elements of a more dynamic and affordable health system. The pace of change, however, will depend on the formation of new alliances among purchasers and motivated providers. By working together, we can accelerate a national commitment to delivering greater value to patients and to society as a whole.

References

Bree Collaborative. 2017. "Accountable Payment Models." Accessed October 11. www.breecollaborative.org/topic-areas/apm/.

de Brantes, F., and K. Love. 2016. "A Process for Structuring Bundled Payments in Maternity Care." *NEJM Catalyst*. Published October 24. http://catalyst.nejm.org/bundled-payments-maternity-care/.

DeVore, B.L., and L. Cates. 2015. "Disruptive Innovation for Healthcare Delivery: Year 1 Report from Intel Corporation and Presbyterian Healthcare Services." Intel Corporation. Accessed October 11, 2017. https://www.intel.com/content/dam/www/public/us/en/documents/white-papers/healthcare-presbyterian-paper.pdf.

Evans, M. 2015. "Boeing Negotiates Directly with More Health Systems." *Modern Healthcare*. Published August 4. www.modernhealthcare.com/article/20150804/NEWS/150809961.

Health Care Payment Learning & Action Network. 2016. *Accelerating and Aligning Clinical Episode Payment Models*. Accessed October 11, 2017. http://hcp-lan.org/workproducts/cep-whitepaper-final.pdf.

Heartland Institute. 2016. "Attachment 7 to Covered California 2017 Individual Market QHP Issuer Contract: Quality, Network Management, Delivery System Standards and Improvement Strategy." Published April 5. www.heartland.org/_template-assets/documents/publications/2017_qhp_issuer_contract_attachment_7_individual_4-5-2016_clean_v3.pdf.

Johns Hopkins Medicine. 2015. "Companies Pay for Employees' Surgeries at Johns Hopkins." *Managed Care Partners*. Published Winter. www.hopkinsmedicine.org/news/publications/managed_care_partners/managed_care_partners_winter_2015/companies_pay_for_employees_surgeries_at_johns_hopkins.

Mecklenburg, R.S. 2016. "A Better Way for Employers to Procure Health Care." *Harvard Business Review*. Published November 17. https://hbr.org/2016/11/a-better-way-for-employers-to-procure-health-care.

National Alliance of Healthcare Purchaser Coalitions. 2017. "Welcome to the National Alliance." Accessed October 11. http://nationalalliancehealth.org/.

Porter, M.E., and T.H. Lee. 2013. "The Strategy That Will Fix Health Care." *Harvard Business Review*. Published October. https://hbr.org/2013/10/the-strategy-that-will-fix-health-care.

Slotkin, J.R., O.A. Ross, M.R. Coleman, and J. Ryu. 2017. "Why GE, Boeing, Lowe's, and Walmart Are Directly Buying Health Care for Employees." *Harvard Business Review*. Published June 8. https://hbr.org/2017/06/why-ge-boeing-lowes-and-walmart-are-directly-buying-health-care-for-employees.

Stapleton, S.R., C. Osborne, and J. Illuzzi. 2013. "Outcomes of Care in Birth Centers: Demonstration of a Durable Model." *Journal of Midwifery & Women's Health* 58 (1): 3–14.

Woo, V.G., T. Lundeen, S. Matula, and A. Milstein. 2017. "Achieving Higher-Value Obstetrical Care." *American Journal of Obstetrics & Gynecology* 216 (3): 250.e1–250.e14.

Zeltner, B. 2012. "Walmart to Send Employees to Cleveland Clinic for Heart Care." Cleveland.com. Published October 12. www.cleveland.com/healthfit/index.ssf/2012/10/wal-mart_to_send_employees_to.html.

Provider-Sponsored Plans: Current Trends and Strategic Implications for Hospitals and Health Systems

by Paul H. Keckley, PhD

Since its passage in 2010, the Affordable Care Act has been the focus of attention for healthcare leaders and strategists, especially as it relates to health insurance and provider payments (see box on page 46). These two areas of reform, coupled with the growing prevalence of and costs associated with chronic disease, have forced hospitals and health systems to rethink their strategies around patient care and place greater emphasis on managing population health and assuming risk for results. In consequence, some have decided to sponsor their own health insurance plans.

Consider the following:

- The number of provider-sponsored plans (PSPs) increased 5 percent from 2015 to 2016 (from 256 plans to 268), and enrollment grew nearly 11 percent, from 32.8 million to 36.3 million. Notably, healthcare information company AIS Health found a shift from group coverage to individual membership, which rose almost 4 percent to 16.7 million (Niranjan 2016).
- An increasing number of healthcare organizations that operate PSPs are providing management and other support services to hospitals and health systems that are launching plans via joint operating agreements.
- Private insurers have created numerous partnerships with hospitals through joint ventures and joint operating agreements to establish PSPs.

Research on PSP Effectiveness

A few recent studies have probed the effectiveness of PSPs, with the majority showing mixed results to date at a substantial cost to their organizations:

- A Robert Wood Johnson Foundation analysis of the 2015–2016 performance of 145 PSPs found that few had adequate enrollment to achieve economies of scale and make a sustainable impact in their local markets. Of the 37 PSPs started after 2010, only 4 were profitable, 5 had gone out of business, and 2 were in the process of being sold (Baumgarten 2017).
- A comparison of 24 PSPs that had top-quartile cash flow and balance sheet stability in 2011–2013 with 72 PSPs in the bottom quartile found that aggressive management of medical costs (as measured by medical loss ratios) was associated with stronger financial performance. Among the best-performing PSPs, medical loss ratios increased from 83.5 percent to 86.4 percent and profit margin ratios slipped from 2.5 percent to 0.4 percent. Providers that avoided declines did so by paying their hospitals and physicians less and

About the Author

Paul H. Keckley, PhD, is managing editor of *The Keckley Report*, a weekly blog covering health industry trends and issues, and an adviser to integrated health systems on strategies for growth and sustainability. He is also a columnist for *Hospitals & Health Networks* magazine and a frequent contributor to healthcare media coverage. Keckley serves on the board of directors for Tivity Health and on advisory boards for the Lipscomb University College of Pharmacy, Western Governors University, the American Association for Physician Leadership, and the American Hospital Association. In 2009, he served as the facilitator for the White House Office of Health Reform in discussions with the major health industry trade associations as the Affordable Care Act was being deliberated. He earned a bachelor's degree at Lipscomb University and master's and doctoral degrees at The Ohio State University, and he completed a graduate fellowship at Oxford University in England.

Provider Health Plans

How likely is it that the following will happen by 2023?

Very Likely (%)	Somewhat Likely (%)	Neutral (%)	Somewhat Unlikely (%)	Very Unlikely (%)
23	13	16	19	29

Your hospital or health system will have been licensed to sell its own health insurance products.

50		30	8	8	4

Your hospital or health system will expand its employment of physician extenders (e.g., nurse practitioners, advanced practice nurses) by at least 50 percent to accommodate demand.

9	22	22	29	18

Your hospital or health system will have a negative gross operating margin for inpatient and outpatient care.

24	29	25	14	8

Your hospital or health system will have included experts in healthcare financing on its governing board.

12	36	28	17	7

Your hospital's or health system's non–patient care revenue (e.g., retail health initiatives, alternative healthcare programs, wellness activities) from commercial insurers, Medicare, and Medicaid will increase 5 percent annually.

Note: Percentages in each row may not sum exactly to 100% because of rounding.

What Hospital Executives Anticipate by 2023

- Relatively few respondents expect their hospital or health system to sell its own insurance products. While 36 percent think this is somewhat to very likely, 48 percent say it is somewhat to very unlikely.

- The vast majority of leaders expect to expand employment of physician extenders by at least 50 percent. Half of respondents (50 percent) believe this is very likely, and another 30 percent say it is somewhat likely.

continued on pg. 46

Key Ways the Affordable Care Act Affects Providers

- **Health insurance.** The law requires individuals and employers to purchase coverage or pay a penalty. It provides for expansion of Medicaid coverage for those under 138 percent of the federal poverty level, as well as subsidized coverage for individuals and small businesses through state-operated health exchanges. Among other key changes, the law also requires that benefits be standardized and that private insurers cover those with preexisting conditions.

- **Provider payments.** The Affordable Care Act shifted provider Medicare and Medicaid payments from fee-for-service to performance-based compensation. It promoted accountable care organizations, bundled payments, value-based payments, patient-centered medical homes, and other mechanisms to increasingly tie reimbursement to outcome, safety, efficiency, and patient experience measures.

—continued from pg. 44

keeping premiums low to maintain adequate enrollment (McCue 2015).

- The American Hospital Association studied the operational, financial, and member experiences of wholly owned PSPs in 50 markets compared to their biggest competitors for that same time period (2011 to 2013). The analysis found that PSPs, including those with the largest enrollments, had worse financial performance than their competitors as measured by median and mean cost-to-premium ratios for Medicare, Medicaid, and commercial insurance. Closely related, the data showed that utilization rates for inpatient and outpatient services were higher for PSPs, a key predictor of their medical costs. Provider plans did outperform other plans in member satisfaction and National Committee for Quality Assurance measures, but insurance is price driven; sponsorship by a local system or access to a wider network of regional providers does not translate to a market advantage for a PSP if premiums are higher than other options accessible to purchasers. The report concluded, "PSPs with larger enrollments perform better than plans with lower enrollments. In general, small enrollments correlate to operating losses, high administrative costs, and poor financial performance" (American Hospital Association 2015).

From these studies, it is clear that successful PSPs have large enrollments, low administrative costs, and aggressive utilization controls, but fewer than one in ten enjoy this advantage.

Implications for Healthcare Leaders

As market forces and the Affordable Care Act push providers to assume financial risk and offer population health management services, many healthcare finance experts believe sponsorship of an insurance plan is the best way to respond. And although the number of these plans is on the rise, the majority of hospital and health system leaders remain skeptical. Only 35 percent of executives responding to the latest *Futurescan* national survey say they are at least somewhat likely to "be licensed to sell" their own insurance product within the next five years, versus 48 percent who say they are very or somewhat unlikely to do so.

I believe the reasons for this reluctance are twofold:

1. **Strategic risks.** The variable historical performance of PSPs and the financial risks associated with operating a successful plan need careful review. For hospitals and health systems that have strong market positions, the opportunity is greater, especially if they are able to use their plan as a hedge against private insurers on premiums and plan design. But might a provider be better served by deploying its capital on revenue growth and program expansion? Might a better path to risk sharing be a joint venture with private insurers or positioning oneself as the leader in delivering high-quality, low-cost care? These are the questions senior executives and boards of directors are asking. For those that choose to sponsor a plan, mitigating these risks requires achieving scale (i.e., 300,000 or more commercial-equivalent lives), managing medical costs aggressively, and offering plans with premiums that are the same as or lower than those of other plans in their market.

continued from pg. 45

- More than half (53 percent) say it is at least somewhat likely their organization's governing board will include experts in healthcare finance.

- Only 31 percent of respondents think it is somewhat to very likely their hospital or health system will have a negative gross operating margin, while 47 percent say this is somewhat to very unlikely.

2. **Regulatory questions.** Uncertainty around the future of health insurance and the regulatory environment at the state and federal levels is a legitimate concern for hospitals and health systems. The major investor-owned plans (United, Anthem, Aetna, Cigna, Humana) and the Blues have gained muscle at the expense of smaller plans and cooperatives. Moreover, the margins in insurance have shrunk, prompting many to exit markets altogether. Providers must be attentive to changes in the regulatory landscape and be prepared to act accordingly.

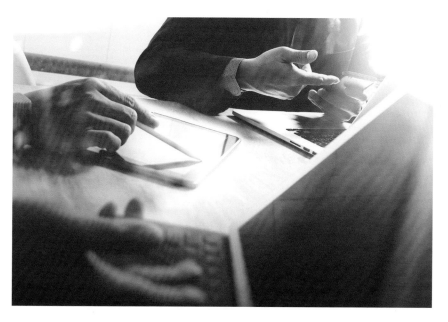

The reality is that hospital and health system margins will be under intense pressure from all purchasers—patients, employers, Medicaid, and Medicare. Deciding whether to sponsor a plan, or how to stabilize a plan that is underperforming, requires careful planning by healthcare leaders:

- For organizations that already sponsor plans, the focus will be on enrollment growth and benefit design innovation, with special attention given to contracting opportunities in Medicaid and Medicare. However, their premiums must be competitive.

- For those in markets where sponsorship makes sense—where unnecessary utilization and avoidable costs are high, the scale and scope of the hospitals' services are adequate to support large-scale population health management, and retaliation by private insurers is not a major concern—there are multiple avenues to proceed with a PSP strategy.
- For those in markets where sponsoring a PSP does not make sense, participation in shared-risk arrangements with payers will be increasingly important. Optimal performance in these alternative payment programs will necessitate investments in care coordination, tightening of physician and post-acute care networks, and surveillance of insurer actions that might enhance or destabilize long-term viability.

For most hospitals and health systems, partnering with another organization makes sense if sponsoring a plan is a desirable strategy. It is not for every organization, but certainly worth considering if circumstances suggest there is opportunity.

References

American Hospital Association. 2015. "The Performance of Provider-Sponsored Health Plans: Key Findings, Strategic Implications." Advocacy issues report. Published October 29. www.aha.org/content/15/pshpreport.pdf.

Baumgarten, A. 2017. "Analysis of Integrated Delivery Systems and New Provider-Sponsored Health Plans." Robert Wood Johnson Foundation. Published June. www.rwjf.org/content/dam/farm/reports/reports/2017/rwjf437615.

McCue, M.J. 2015. "Assessing the Financial Condition of Provider-Sponsored Health Plans." *Managed Care* 24 (6): 39–44.

Niranjan, N. 2016. "AIS Shows Growth in Provider-Sponsored Plans and Individual Market." GetInsured. Published June 30. https://company.getinsured.com/resources/blog/ais-shows-growth-in-provider-sponsored-plans-and-individual-market/.

ABOUT THE CONTRIBUTORS

Society for Healthcare Strategy & Market Development

Executive director: Diane Weber, RN
Senior editorial specialist: Brian Griffin
Research data analytics specialist: Ann Feeney

The Society for Healthcare Strategy & Market Development of the American Hospital Association is the largest and most prominent voice for healthcare strategists in planning, marketing, communications, public relations, business development, and physician strategy.

SHSMD is committed to leading, connecting, and serving its members to prepare them for the future with greater knowledge and opportunity as their organizations strive to improve the health of their communities. The society provides a broad and constantly updated array of resources, services, experiences, and connections.

SHSMD leaders are available for on-site presentations about *Futurescan 2018–2023* to healthcare governing boards, senior management, planning teams, and medical staffs. To arrange for a presentation, contact SHSMD at 312.422.3888 or shsmd@aha.org.

American College of Healthcare Executives/Health Administration Press

President and CEO: Deborah J. Bowen, FACHE, CAE
Director, Health Administration Press: Michael E. Cunningham, CAE
Project manager: Andrew J. Baumann
Layout editor: Cepheus Edmondson

The American College of Healthcare Executives is an international professional society of 40,000 healthcare executives who lead hospitals, healthcare systems and other healthcare organizations. ACHE's mission is to advance its members and healthcare management excellence. ACHE offers its prestigious FACHE® credential, signifying board certification in healthcare management. ACHE's established network of 78 chapters provides access to networking, education and career development at the local level. In addition, ACHE is known for its magazine, *Healthcare Executive*, and its career development and public policy programs. Through such efforts, ACHE works toward its vision of being the preeminent professional society for leaders dedicated to improving health.

The Foundation of the American College of Healthcare Executives was established to further advance healthcare management excellence through education and research. The Foundation of ACHE is known for its educational programs—including the annual Congress on Healthcare Leadership, which draws more than 4,000 participants—and groundbreaking research. Its publishing division, Health Administration Press, is one of the largest publishers of books and journals on health services management, including textbooks for college and university courses. For more information, visit www.ache.org.

ABOUT THE SPONSOR

The American Hospital Association is a not-for-profit association of health care provider organizations and individuals that are committed to the improvement of health in their communities. The AHA is the national advocate for its members, which include nearly 5,000 hospitals, health care systems, networks and other providers of care. Founded in 1898, the AHA provides education for health care leaders and is a source of information on health care issues and trends. For more information, visit www.aha.org.